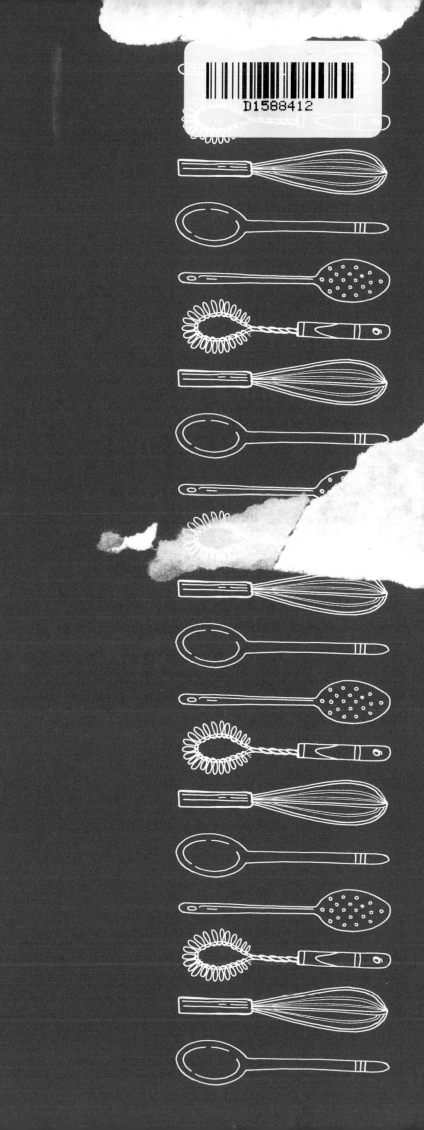

THE FOODS THAT HEAL
COOKBOOK

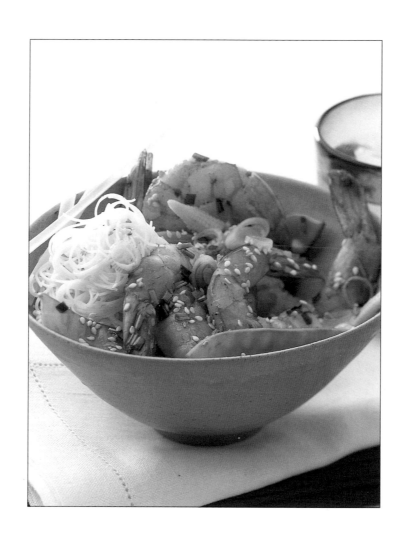

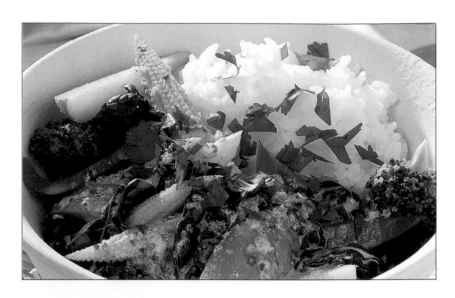

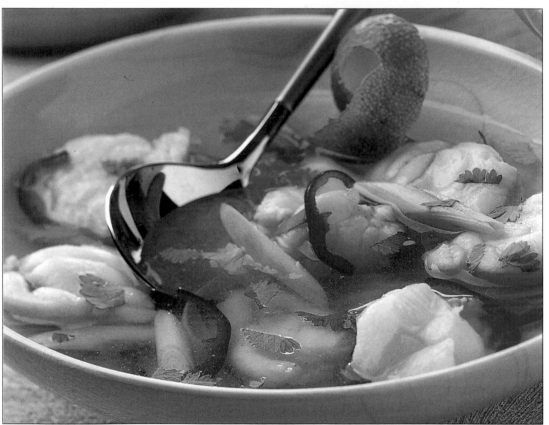

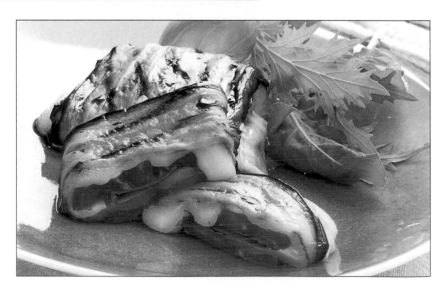

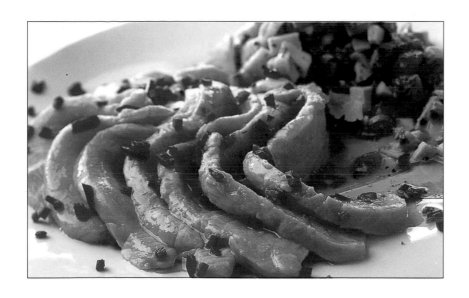

THE FOODS THAT HEAL
COOKBOOK

OVER 50 DELICIOUS RECIPES
FOR HEALING THE BODY

NICOLA GRAIMES

LORENZ BOOKS

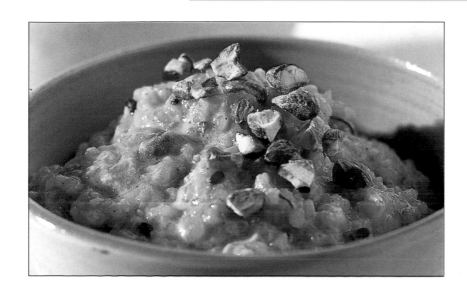

First published in 2000 by Lorenz Books

© Anness Publishing Limited 2000

Lorenz Books is an imprint of
Anness Publishing Limited
Hermes House
88–89 Blackfriars Road
London SE1 8HA

This edition distributed in Canada by Raincoast Books
8680 Cambie Street, Vancouver, British Columbia V6P 6M9

Publisher: Joanna Lorenz
Executive Editor: Linda Fraser
Project Editor: Susannah Blake
Editorial Reader: Joy Wotton
Photographers: Janine Hosegood (introduction) and Thomas Odulate (recipes);
p6, p7t, p7b, p8 and p9t Tony Stone Images; p9b Superstock
Designer: Nigel Partridge
Nutritional Consultant: Clare Brain
Indexer: Hilary Bird
Production Controller: Don Campaniello

1 3 5 7 9 10 8 6 4 2

NOTES
For all recipes, quantities are given in both metric and imperial measures
and, where appropriate, measures are also given in standard cups and spoons.
Follow one set, but not a mixture, because they are not interchangeable.

Standard spoon and cup measures are level.
1 tsp = 5ml, 1 tbsp = 15ml, 1 cup = 250ml/8fl oz

Australian standard tablespoons are 20ml. Australian readers should
use 3 tsp in place of 1 tbsp for measuring small quantities

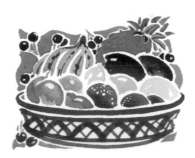

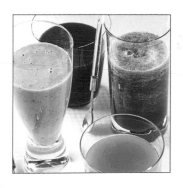

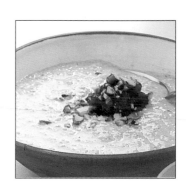

CONTENTS

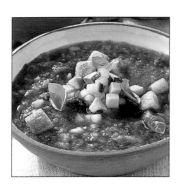

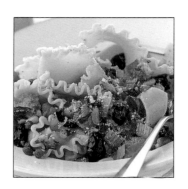

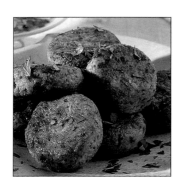

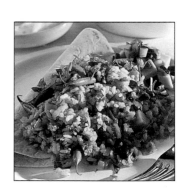

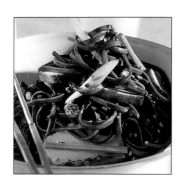

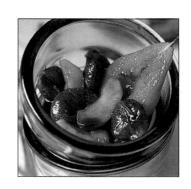

Introduction

A growing interest in the impact of nutrition on health, combined with improved research methods, has enabled scientists to look more closely at the health benefits of foods. It is more apparent than ever that what we eat has a huge influence on our health, and strong links between poor diet and many serious diseases have been made.

We now know that there is a strong link between poor nutrition and both cancer and heart disease. Numerous studies have revealed that food is much more than fuel; many foods are believed to have great health benefits and therapeutic properties, while others can have negative effects. With this knowledge we now have the opportunity to follow the healthiest possible diet.

A NATURAL PHARMACY

One of the most exciting developments in recent years has been the discovery of plant compounds called phytochemicals, which are found in vegetables, fruit, grains, nuts and seeds. There are literally thousands of these naturally occurring compounds and, although research is still at an early stage, many scientists suggest that these chemicals could offer a staggering range of health benefits. Phytochemicals are believed to offer protection against some kinds of cancer, heart disease, cataracts, osteoporosis, diabetes and strokes.

Eating more fruit and vegetables is not difficult, yet this simple step is seen as one of the most positive ways of promoting good health. It may even be more important than reducing our intake of saturated fats and processed foods, although this still remains high on the agenda. The presence of phytochemicals – and their benefits – has been hailed as a major nutritional discovery, and we are likely to hear a great deal more about their importance to our health and general well-being in the future.

POLLUTION AND STRESS

In a world that is becoming increasingly polluted, and where individuals are subject to more and more stress, it is all too easy for our bodies to become out of kilter, and for normal bodily functions and processes to be disrupted. Researchers are particularly interested in the role of essential fatty acids, especially those found in oily fish and antioxidants (compounds which help to reduce cell damage).

Antioxidant compounds, such as betacarotene, vitamins C and E, selenium and zinc, to name but a few, are found in fruit and vegetables, as well as wholegrain cereals, nuts, pulses and seeds. As with phytochemicals, it is thought that these antioxidants can reduce the risks of, and fight against, many of the major diseases that affect people in the West. According to certain experts, antioxidants may, in some instances, be even more efficacious than drugs. More research is being carried out all the time to increase our knowledge and understanding of this area.

Below: Eating plenty of fruit and vegetables is an easy way of ensuring a regular intake of valuable health-giving phytochemicals.

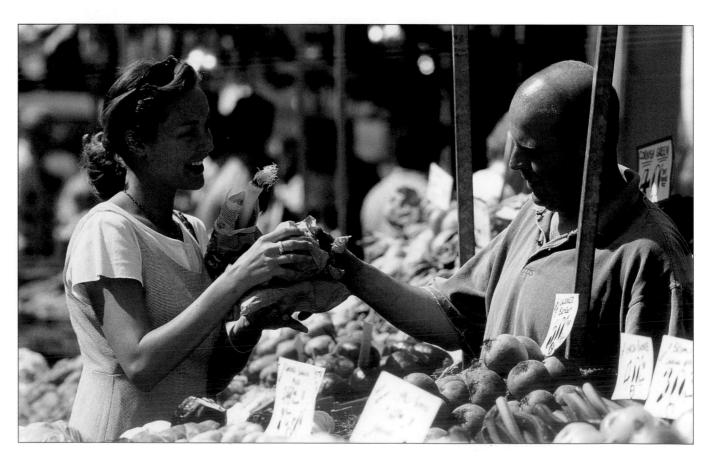

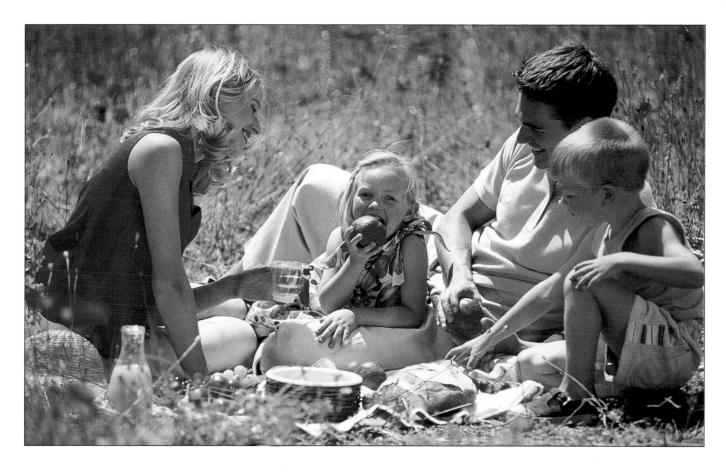

FOODS THAT HEAL

The foods that are believed to offer specific health benefits have become known as "healing foods". However, it is important to accept that while they have a great deal to offer, common sense should prevail. Just because carrots, for example, are good for us does not mean that we should eat excessive quantities of them every day. What really matters is

Below: Naturally grown foods, such as fruit and vegetables, are packed with compounds that can help to fight disease.

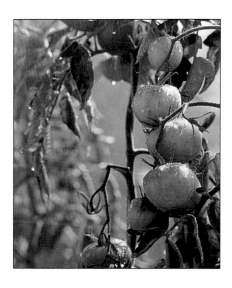

that "healing foods" are part of a diet that is intrinsically balanced, and which also gives us pleasure. Painstaking monitoring of what we eat is not necessary, since this can sap our enjoyment of food.

AN HISTORICAL PERSPECTIVE

Although this book concentrates on the latest research, the idea that food can provide therapeutic benefits is hardly new. Every culture throughout history has used food to prevent illness and boost health. In fact, there was probably little distinction between food and medicine in the distant past. The ancient Egyptians praised the lentil for its ability to lighten the mind; the ancient Greeks and Romans used honey to heal wounds; in ancient China, sprouted beans and grains were used to treat a wide range of health conditions, from constipation to dropsy, while ginger was recommended for joint problems.

Herbs and spices have been revered for thousands of years for their medicinal properties. The ancient Egyptians valued camomile above all other herbs, hailing it as the elixir of youth. They also had high regard for coriander, and seeds of this spice have been found in the tombs of the

Above: Enjoying a varied and well-balanced diet, which is rich in fruits and vegetables, is essential for good health.

pharaohs. More recently, cinnamon and ginger were recommended for sickness and headaches, and feverfew was used in the 18th century to treat migraines.

ABOUT THIS BOOK

In the chapters that follow, you will find information on the healing properties of foods and advice on which of those foods you should include in your diet if you have a particular illness or specific condition. This information is based on the latest research and aims to arm you with the means to make decisions and make positive changes to your diet.

Seeking Professional Advice

It is important to seek professional advice from a doctor, nutritionist, state registered dietitian or medical specialist before making any major changes to your diet. Certain foods may improve a particular condition in some, but may have a negative effect in others.

A Healthy Balance

We are often told to eat a balanced diet, but are unsure of what this actually means. The key to good health is a varied diet that provides the correct proportions of carbohydrate, fibre, protein, fat and vitamins and minerals, as well as water.

The ideal diet includes sufficient calories to provide the body with energy and the nutrients for daily life. It also provides the nutrients and energy needed to combat illness and disease. Getting this balance right is crucial for good health.

Even if you have a condition for which specific foods are suggested, your first priority should still be to take an overview of your general diet. By ensuring that you eat the correct balance of different foods, you will give your body every opportunity to take advantage of the benefits healing foods can bring.

MAKING THE RIGHT CHOICES
Starchy Carbohydrates

This group of foods includes breakfast cereals, bread, rice, pasta, noodles and potatoes, and is essential for a healthy balanced diet. Starchy carbohydrates should make up around 35–40 per cent of what we eat every day. These foods should form the largest part of every meal since they supply the body with the sustained energy that it needs to function effectively. These foods are naturally low in fat and high in fibre. They also provide the body with useful amounts of B vitamins and minerals. Whenever possible, try to choose wholemeal or wholegrain varieties as these are richer in fibre and nutrients, and help to protect against digestive disorders and heart disease.

Fruit and Vegetables

Aim to eat at least five servings of fruit and vegetables a day – a serving is equivalent to one medium apple, banana or orange, a handful of cherry tomatoes, a wine glass of fresh fruit juice, two or more heaped serving spoonfuls of cooked vegetables or a bowl of salad. Choose a wide variety of fresh produce. Fruit and vegetables contain significant amounts of phytochemicals, vitamins, minerals and fibre, and they are low in fat and calories. Cruciferous vegetables, such as broccoli, cabbage, Brussels sprouts, cauliflower and chard, provide plenty of antioxidants, which are believed to protect against certain cancers and heart disease. Bright orange, yellow and red fruit and vegetables, including carrots, sweet potatoes, swede, mangoes, oranges and strawberries, are rich in the antioxidants betacarotene and vitamin C, and they are believed to reduce the risk of heart disease and certain cancers as well.

Meat, Fish and Protein Alternatives

It is recommended that we include a moderate amount of lean meat and poultry, fish, eggs, pulses, tofu and nuts in our diet – around two to three different types a day. Limit red meat to three to four servings a week, an average serving being 115g/4oz–175g/6oz. Eat oily fish, such as herring, sardines, mackerel, salmon and tuna, at least twice a week. These fish contain rich supplies of omega-3 fatty acids, which are thought to help reduce the risk of heart disease. Limit egg intake to three a week. All these foods provide valuable amounts of protein, fibre, iron, calcium, zinc, and vitamins B and E.

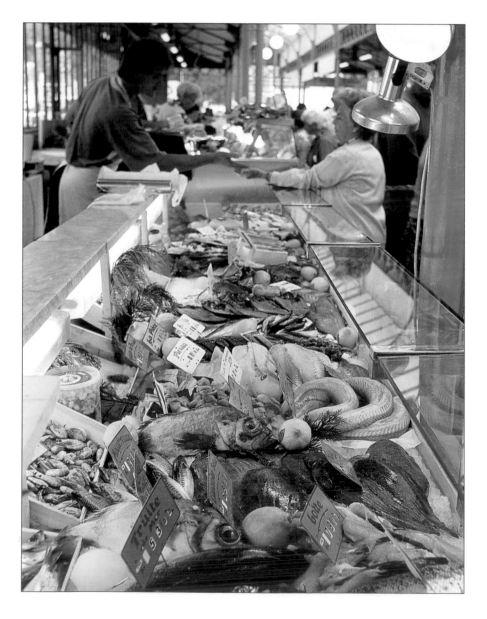

Left: Making a few simple changes to your diet, such as deciding to eat more oily fish, can help to provide your body with the nutrients it needs to sustain good health.

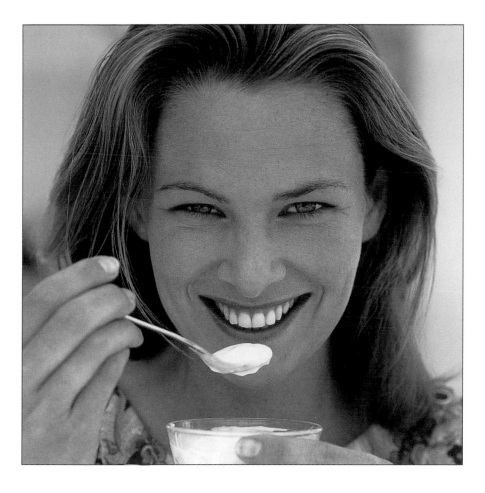

Water

While water plays a vital role in the body, few of us drink enough of it. The average adult requires at least 2.5 litres/4 pints/ 2½ US quarts of liquid a day, and water is the best choice. Tea, coffee and many fizzy drinks contain caffeine and also have a diuretic effect, so that they actually tend to dehydrate the body. It is better to choose herbal teas, natural coffee substitutes and freshly squeezed fruit juices instead.

Left: Consuming three portions of milk, cheese or yogurt a day will provide valuable amounts of protein and calcium as well as supplying essential vitamins and minerals.

Below: Water is one of the keystones of good health, and adults should drink at least eight glasses of water every day.

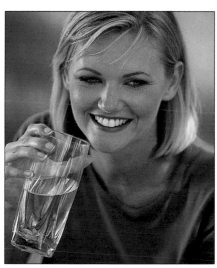

Dairy Produce

Try to eat about three servings of milk, cheese and yogurt a day. These foods provide valuable amounts of protein and calcium, as well as vitamins B_{12}, A and D, which are essential for healthy teeth and bones. Dairy produce can be high in fat, so opt for low-fat varieties and eat them in moderation – a serving is equivalent to 300ml/½ pint/1¼ cups milk, 25g/1oz cheese or a small pot of yogurt.

High-fat and High-sugar Foods

This diverse group of foods includes crisps, chocolate, cakes and biscuits, as well as processed foods. They provide very few nutrients, are laden with calories, and may contribute to malnutrition, weight gain and tooth decay. Try to eat them only occasionally as a treat. Alcohol comes into the same category. High in calories but with little nutritional value, it should be drunk only in moderation.

How to Preserve Nutrients

The general advice throughout this book is to eat plenty of fresh produce and to avoid all heavily processed foods. The nutrients in fresh food, particularly fruit and vegetables, can be unstable and are vulnerable to damage from prolonged storage, incorrect methods of preparation and overcooking. The following tips will help you to get the most value from your food.

• Buy fruits and vegetables that are as fresh as possible and purchase them in small quantities, which you will be able to use quickly. Also buy from suppliers

or shops that have a rapid turnover of produce so that you know it is fresh.

• Avoid fresh produce stored under fluorescent lighting as this can set off a chemical reaction that depletes nutrients.

• Buy organic fruit and vegetables, where possible. Avoid peeling them, as valuable nutrients are stored just below the skin. Instead, simply wash them thoroughly.

• Do not prepare fruit and vegetables too far in advance of serving, as nutrients, such as vitamin C, begin to diminish after cutting and peeling.

• Avoid boiling fruits and vegetables as this destroys the water-soluble vitamin C

and B vitamins. Try to eat some raw fruit and vegetables every day. If you must cook them, use a steamer, since this method of cooking does not have such a detrimental effect on nutrients as methods such as boiling.

• Buy nuts and seeds in small quantities from a supplier with a fast turnover of produce and try to use them up quickly. Store them in airtight containers, in a cool, dark place, or they may become rancid. Herbs, spices, pulses, flours and grains should be kept in the same way.

• Store oils in a cool, dark place to prevent oxidation.

Phytochemicals

Recent research has identified a vast number of natural plant compounds that may play a crucial role in preventing cancer, heart disease, arthritis, diabetes, hypertension and many other health problems. These compounds are collectively known as phytochemicals, and, in the future, they may be classed as essential nutrients.

Everyone knows that fruits, vegetables, grains, nuts and seeds are an essential part of a healthy diet, but they could be even more important than previously thought. While it is true that fresh produce plays a crucial part in our diet because it provides health-promoting antioxidants such as betacarotene, vitamin C and E, this is just part of the picture.

Before phytochemicals were isolated, the chemicals in fruits and vegetables were more broadly classified as vitamins, but scientists have now categorized these plant compounds into groups based on the protective functions they share as well as physical and chemical characteristics.

Scientists have identified thousands of plant compounds, all of which have specific health benefits. The following are just a handful of these extraordinary compounds and their health-giving properties. To get the most from phytochemicals, we should eat at least five types of vegetables and fruit a day, plus wholegrains, pulses, nuts and seeds.

Below: Soya beans and products made from them, such as tofu, contain isoflavones. They are thought to lower blood cholesterol levels.

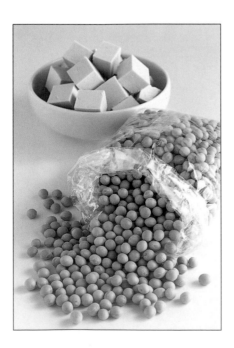

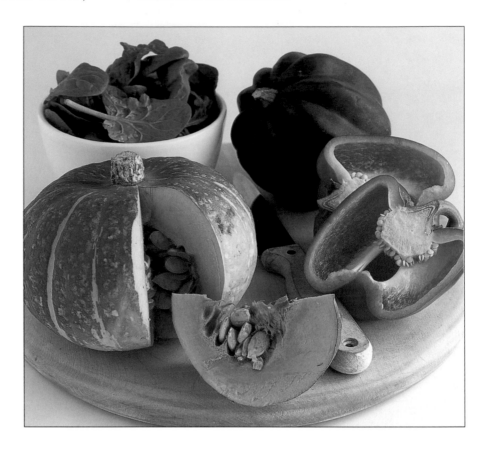

Above: Carotenoids are found in spinach and yellow, orange and red fruit and vegetables, such as pumpkin, squash and red peppers.

PHYTOESTROGENS

In Japan, the symptoms associated with the menopause, such as hot flushes and osteoporosis, are virtually unheard of. This has been attributed to a diet high in soya products, which contain isoflavones. These belong to a group of compounds called phytoestrogens, which have a structure similar to that of the female hormone oestrogen. Isoflavones may also protect against breast, bowel and prostate cancer and help to lower blood cholesterol levels, thereby reducing the risk of heart disease and strokes. Lignans are another phyto-estrogen, which are found in wholegrains, linseeds and berries, and may help to protect against hormone-related cancers.

There are a large number of soya products available that contain valuable isoflavones, including tofu (beancurd), textured vegetable protein (TVP), tempeh, beancurd skins and sticks, and soya milk. It is recommended that women should eat one of these foods every day.

CAROTENOIDS

There are over 600 naturally occurring carotenoids, of which the orange pigment betacarotene is the best known. They are believed to have anti-carcinogenic properties and may also reduce the risk of heart disease, strokes and cataracts.

Betacarotene is found in carrots, peppers, oranges, pink grapefruit and sweet potatoes. Lycopene, a red pigment, is another carotenoid and can be found in tomatoes and tomato products, and also in watermelon, pink grapefruit and canned apricots. Processing seems to increase the availability of lycopene, so more is present in canned and puréed tomatoes. Studies have shown that the compound can reduce the risk of certain cancers, including breast, prostate, colon, stomach and lung cancer, as well as heart disease.

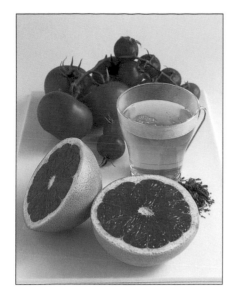

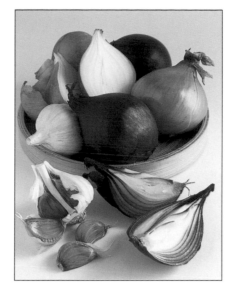

Above: The red pigment, lycopene, which is found in tomatoes, pink grapefruit and green tea, is thought to reduce the risk of some cancers, including colon, stomach and lung.

Above: Alliums, especially onions and garlic, have long been valued for their healing properties, including their antibacterial and antiviral qualities.

FLAVONOIDS

These are part of the plant polyphenol class of phytochemicals. Flavonoids are found in most fruits, vegetables and soya products, and are believed to promote the body's absorption of vitamin C. Research has now shown that these phytochemicals may have quite broad health benefits, such as acting against some cancers, allergies, ulcers, viruses and cataracts, reducing high blood pressure and boosting the immune system.

This group also features a group of compounds called flavonols, which includes quercetin, a phytochemical that is found in apples, onions, black tea, red wine, potatoes and grapes. Research shows that flavonols may help to reduce the risk of heart disease and strokes.

Green tea provides another flavonoid, catechins, which has anti-carcinogenic properties. In countries, such as Japan, where the consumption of green tea is very high, the cancer rates are relatively low. Green tea is also thought to protect against heart disease.

GLUCOSINOLATES

This group of compounds provides an anti-carcinogenic cocktail including indoles and isothiocyanates, which are thought to play a crucial role in fighting disease by stimulating the body's enzyme defences against cancer-inducing substances. Recent studies have shown that 67 per cent of people who ate a diet that was rich in glucosinolates were less likely to succumb to cancer.

Cruciferous vegetables, such as broccoli, cabbage, Brussels sprouts, kale, pak choi, watercress, turnips, cauliflower and swede, are an excellent source of this group of valuable phytochemicals.

ALLIUM COMPOUNDS

These compounds are found in the plants belonging to the genus *Allium*. Garlic and onions are the most potent members of this family of vegetables, which includes leeks, shallots, spring onions and chives.

These contain allicin sulphides, which are thought to reduce the risk of cancer and boost heart health. They are released when the plant is cut open and are the chemicals responsible for making the eyes water when chopping onions.

As well as fighting cancer and promoting heart function, allium compounds are believed to help to reduce blood cholesterol levels, lower blood pressure and inhibit blood clotting, which can lead to strokes. These compounds may also activate and promote liver detoxification and appear to have potent antiviral and antibacterial qualities.

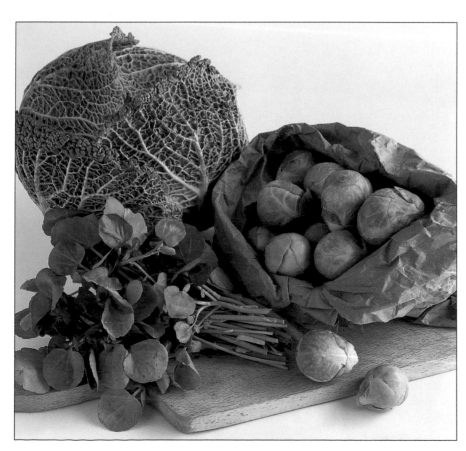

Left: Cruciferous vegetables, such as Savoy cabbage, Brussels sprouts and watercress, contain rich supplies of the cancer-fighting phytochemicals, glucosinolates.

Essential Nutrients

A healthy diet is a balanced diet. There are four key elements to a balanced diet – carbohydrates, fibre, protein and fat – which provide essential vitamins and minerals. If these are consumed in the correct proportions, they will provide the body with long-term energy and the balance of nutrients that is needed to maintain good health.

CARBOHYDRATES

Until quite recently starchy foods received a bad press. They were blamed for making us fat, and many low-carbohydrate and carbohydrate-free diets were developed. It is now recognized that they are the body's major source of energy and an essential part of a healthy diet. They are vital if our bodies are to function properly.

Carbohydrate foods tend to be lower in fat than other food types, and they are generally more filling because they contain fibre. They are made up of starches, fibre and sugars. The group includes cereals, bread, potatoes, pasta and rice. Whenever possible, choose unrefined carbohydrates, such as wholemeal bread, in preference to refined carbohydrates, such as white bread, as the latter are stripped of many valuable nutrients during processing.

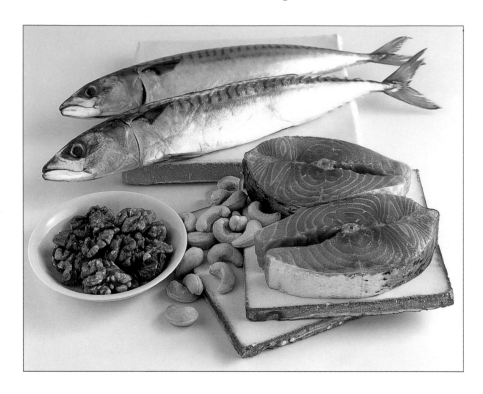

Above: Oily fish, such as mackerel and salmon, and some nuts are a good source of omega-3 fatty acids, which have been found to reduce the risk of heart disease.

FIBRE

Fruit, vegetables, grains, legumes, nuts and seeds are the main source of fibre in our diet. There are two types – insoluble and soluble. Insoluble fibre, found in whole wheat, brown rice, bran and nuts, gives bulk to our food and helps to combat constipation by ensuring that the digestive system functions properly. Soluble fibre, from pulses, fruit, vegetables and oats, binds with toxins in the gut, promoting their excretion. It also helps to reduce blood cholesterol. Eating both types of fibre can reduce the risk of such bowel disorders as diverticulitis, and colon and rectal cancer. However, bran may aggravate the symptoms of irritable bowel syndrome (IBS), so if you suffer from IBS, consult your doctor before making any changes to your diet. As fibre provides bulk in the diet, it will help to reduce hunger pangs – particularly useful for those who are trying to lose weight.

PROTEIN

This is essential for the maintenance and repair of the body's cells, as well as the proper functioning of enzymes, hormones and antibodies. Protein is made up of 22 amino acids. Fourteen of these can be manufactured in the body, but the other eight have to be provided through the diet. A food that contains all eight of these amino acids is said to be a "complete" or "high-quality" protein. Meat, eggs, dairy products and soya beans fall into this category. Protein from plant sources does not usually contain all eight required amino acids, and is therefore known as an "incomplete" protein. Foods within this category are still valuable in the diet and should be incorporated. They include nuts, potatoes, legumes, cereals, rice and pasta.

FATS

Some fat is essential to a healthy diet as it provides vitamins A, D and E, and essential fatty acids the body cannot manufacture. Fat should make up no more than 33 per cent of the diet; the type of fat consumed is as important as the amount.

Saturated fat, which is solid at room temperature, is found mainly in animal products. It has been associated with an increased risk of cancer and coronary heart disease, so it should be eaten in moderation. A simple way to reduce the amount of saturated fat you eat is always to trim meat of any visible fat before cooking and to skin poultry, for example.

Unsaturated fat, both poly- and mono-unsaturated, which is usually liquid at room temperature, is as high in calories as saturated fat; but it offers some health benefits as well. Polyunsaturated fat provides omega-3 and omega-6 essential fatty acids. The consumption of omega-3 fatty acids (linolenic acid), which are found in oily fish, walnuts, soya beans and wheatgerm, has been found to reduce the risk of blood clots, heart disease and strokes. Polyunsaturated fat also helps regulate blood pressure. Omega-6 fatty acids (linoleic acid and their oils), which can be found in nuts and seeds, have been found to reduce blood cholesterol levels. Other key health benefits attributed to omega-3 and omega-6 fatty acids include a reduced risk of arthritis and certain cancers, and a positive effect on various skin complaints, the symptoms of PMS (pre-menstrual syndrome) and the side-effects of the menopause. The benefits of both omega-3 and omega-6 fatty acids are now believed to be even more important than originally thought, and it is important to include a good supply of both types of these fats in your diet.

WATER

The importance of water is often taken for granted. Although it is possible to survive for weeks without food, we can only live a few days without water. It plays a vital role in the body: it transports nutrients, regulates the body temperature, transports waste, and acts as a lubricating fluid. Most people do not drink enough water: it is thought that an adult requires around 2.5litres/ 4 pints/2½ US quarts per day. A shortage of water can provoke headaches and loss of concentration. Fizzy drinks, tea and coffee all act as diuretics and speed up the loss of water, causing dehydration.

VITAMINS AND MINERALS

These nutrients assist in the release of energy and are required in varying quantities depending on state of health, lifestyle and age. Vitamins are either water soluble or fat soluble. The water-soluble B vitamins and vitamin C cannot be stored in the body, so a regular intake is needed. Fat-soluble vitamins A, D, E and K are stored in the liver. There are 16 essential minerals. Some are required in quite large amounts, while trace elements are needed in tiny quantities. Minerals predominantly regulate and balance the body, and help to maintain a healthy immune system.

Antioxidants

These ensure the damage caused to the body's cells by free radicals is kept to a minimum. Free radicals are produced naturally in the body, and as a result of other factors such as pollution and poor diet. They attack the genetic material, held inside the cells, causing it to mutate.

As well as protecting us against the damage caused by free radicals, anti-oxidants stimulate the immune system and normalize the balance of hormone-like chemicals in the body that control pain, inflammation and fever.

Key antioxidant nutrients include vitamins A, C and E and minerals, such as selenium and zinc. Measures we can take to boost our antioxidant levels include:
• Eat foods rich in betacarotene (converted to vitamin A in the body) – found in leafy vegetables and fruit, especially apricots and mangoes, dairy produce, cod liver oil, liver and enriched margarine. Vitamin A is fat soluble, so can be stored in the body.
• Eat plenty of vitamin C-rich foods, such as citrus fruits, green vegetables and wholegrain cereals. Vitamin C is water

soluble, so needs to be replenished as the body flushes out any excess.
• Consume adequate amounts of fat-soluble vitamin E, found in seeds, green leafy vegetables and enriched margarine.
• Include foods that contain the trace elements zinc and selenium. Zinc is found in shellfish, meat, eggs, wholegrain cereals and pulses; selenium in whole-grain cereals, meat and fish.

Below: A diet that contains plenty of fresh fruit and vegetables will provide a good source of protective antioxidants.

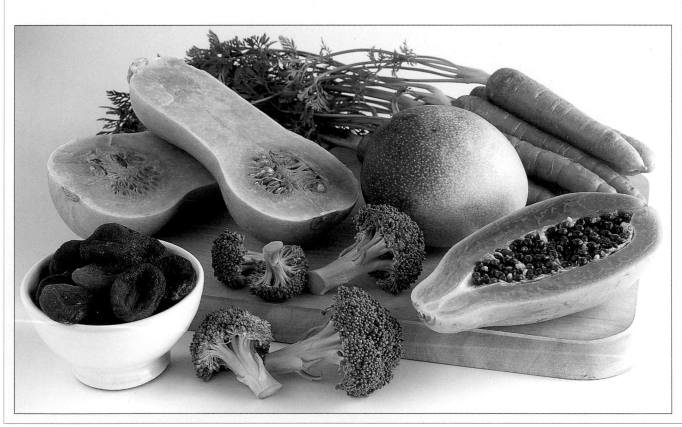

Looking After Your Heart

Despite medical advances and research into diet, coronary heart disease (CHD) still remains the number one killer of both men and women in the Western world. There has been a great deal of debate and controversy recently over the relationship between diet and CHD. Most health experts agree that our dietary habits, as well as lifestyle measures, can help to lessen the risk of a heart attack, lower blood cholesterol and reduce high blood pressure.

KEY PROTECTIVE FOODS

Oily fish Omega-3 fatty acids, which can be found in oily fish, such as tuna, herrings, sardines, mackerel and salmon, along with walnuts, wheatgerm, soya beans, rapeseed oil and linseeds, have been found to play a crucial part in reducing the rate of deaths from heart disease, and also the incidence of non-fatal heart attacks and strokes. As little as one serving of oily fish each week is believed to cut the risk of a heart attack by half. These fatty acids thin the blood and, in turn, help to prevent blood clots and reduce blood cholesterol levels.

Oats, lentils, nuts and pulses These foods provide insoluble fibre, which can reduce blood cholesterol levels when part of a low-fat diet. Oats have also been found to reduce high blood pressure.

Fruits and vegetables These foodstuffs provide soluble fibre (pectin) as well as generous amounts of phytochemicals, antioxidants, vitamins C and E, and betacarotene, which the body converts to vitamin A. They help to prevent the furring-up of the arteries that leads to atherosclerosis and, in addition, support the body's defence system.

Below: Red wine contains quercetin, which is thought to protect against heart disease.

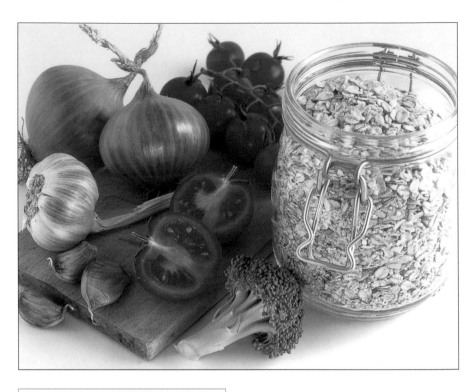

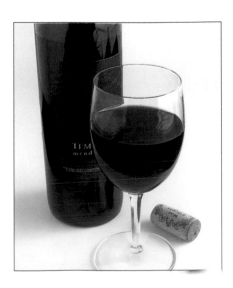

Folic Acid
Foods that are rich in folic acid, including pulses and green vegetables, may help to lower the risk of heart disease by reducing levels of the amino acid, homocysteine. High levels of this amino acid have been linked to an increased risk of coronary heart disease (CHD) and strokes.

Garlic The inclusion of garlic in a balanced diet has been found to lower blood cholesterol levels, reduce blood pressure and help to prevent the formation of blood clots. It has been claimed that eating one or two garlic cloves a day reduces the probability of a second heart attack by half in previous heart patients.

Red wine, apples, tea and onions This disparate group contains the flavonoid quercetin, which research shows may reduce the risk of heart disease and strokes. However, red wine should be drunk only in moderation, and medical advice should be taken first.

Above: Onions, tomatoes, oats, broccoli and garlic may reduce the risk of heart disease.

Soya beans and products These can reduce blood cholesterol levels, if eaten on a regular basis.

FOODS TO AVOID
Cut down on foods that are high in saturated fat, including dairy products, fatty meat, and hydrogenated or trans fats found in margarine and processed foods. Drink alcohol in moderation (if your doctor allows this) and cut down the amount of salt you ingest.

Shopping Essentials
• Oily fish (eat two or three times a week)
• Oats, lentils, nuts and pulses, especially soya beans
• Fruit and vegetables, especially onions, apples and garlic
• Tea and red wine (drink in moderation)

Improving Your Lung Function

The incidence of respiratory problems is increasing every year. These problems may be genetic or they may result from – or be exacerbated by – poor air quality, pollution and cigarette smoke, as well as allergies to animals, dust, pollen, artificial additives and certain foods. Recent studies show that respiratory problems, such as asthma, congested sinuses and catarrh, can often be alleviated by a healthy, balanced diet and by avoiding particular foods, such as wine, dairy products and processed foods. Fruit and vegetables are also key to keeping the lungs and airways in good shape.

KEY PROTECTIVE FOODS

Green vegetables Broccoli, peas, cabbage, spinach and other leafy green vegetables, are a good source of antioxidants, which help to keep airways healthy.

Carrots, sweet potatoes, apricots and mangoes These orange fruits and vegetables provide betacarotene, which may help to prevent inflammation of the lungs and airways.

Citrus fruits, melon, strawberries and kiwi fruit These are rich in vitamin C, which can offer real relief to asthmatics and those suffering from a wide range of other respiratory problems.

Tomatoes and tomato products These are believed to help lower the risk of developing asthma.

Onions These clear the airways and may therefore help to prevent asthma attacks.

Wholegrains, wheatgerm, dried figs, nuts and seeds These are a good source of

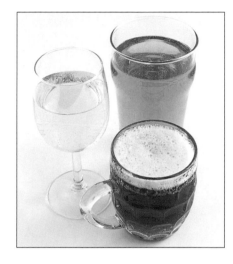

Above: Beer, wine and cider often contain chemicals that can exacerbate breathing problems and should be avoided.

magnesium, which can aid the relaxation of the muscles of the airways.

Sunflower oil and seeds Together with pine nuts, almonds, broccoli, avocados, oats and margarine, sunflower oil and seeds provide the antioxidant vitamin E, which is an anti-inflammatory.

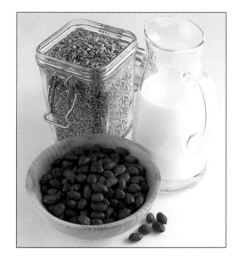

Above: Wheat, nuts and dairy products are common allergens, which may aggravate asthma and sinus problems.

Ginger and chilli These spices can help to thin mucus and relieve congested airways.

Garlic This antiviral and antibacterial allium can also act as a nasal decongestant.

Raw, unfiltered honey This type of honey is often used as a traditional remedy for hay fever sufferers. It can also help to desensitize the airways.

FOODS TO AVOID

Reducing or eliminating wine, beer, cider, salt, dairy products, wheat, food additives, yeast and red meat from your diet may help to alleviate respiratory problems.

Below: Eat plenty of unrefined, unprocessed foods to keep the lungs and airways healthy.

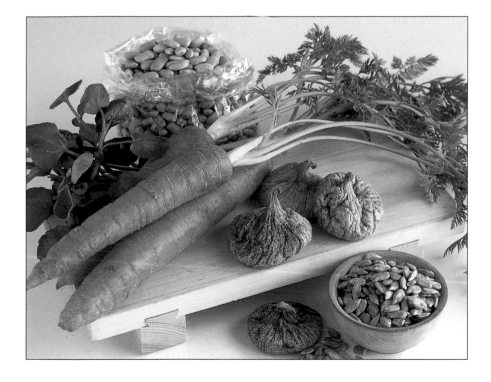

> ### Shopping Essentials
> • Green vegetables, onions, carrots, garlic, tomatoes and sweet potatoes
> • Fruit, especially apricots, mangoes, citrus fruits, melon, strawberries and kiwi fruit
> • Spices, especially ginger and chillies
> • Wholegrains, wheatgerm and oats
> • Dried figs, nuts and seeds
> • Sunflower oil and margarine
> • Raw, unfiltered honey

Boosting Your Immune System

A strong immune system is vital for maintaining general good health and warding off infections. Poor diet and stress are the most common causes of a weakened immune system, leaving the body vulnerable to colds, flu and disease. A diet based on unprocessed foods, as well as a healthy lifestyle, is essential for maintaining the immune system.

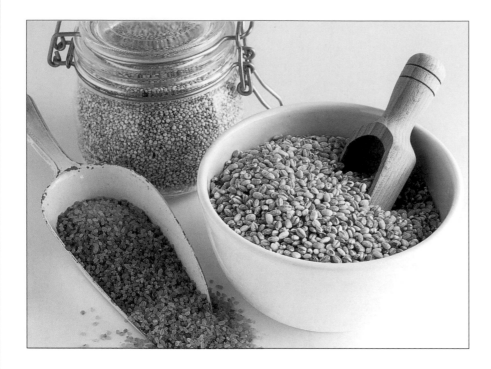

Above: Quinoa, barley and bulgur wheat are rich in vitamin B_6, which helps fight infection.

KEY PROTECTIVE FOODS

Fruit and vegetables Citrus fruits, berries, blackcurrants, sweet potatoes, peppers, green vegetables, carrots and avocados are good sources of the immune-boosting antioxidants, vitamins C and E and betacarotene. Also include nuts and seeds.

Lemons and limes These citrus fruits are good for colds, coughs and sore throats. They are rich in vitamin C and also have potent antiseptic properties.

Below: Garlic and spices, such as chilli, ginger and turmeric, help to fight coughs and colds.

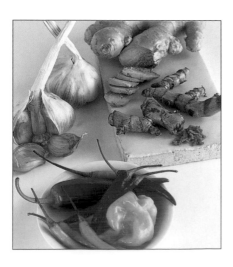

Wholegrains, meat, tuna, salmon, nuts, seeds and bananas These all provide vitamin B_6, which supports the body's production of antibodies. If you have a cold, however, avoid dairy produce, as it is mucus-forming.

Shellfish Oysters and crab provide zinc, which can help to fight against infection. Other sources include eggs, beef, turkey and pumpkin seeds.

Chicken, watercress and raspberries These foods are said to be effective in breaking down mucus.

Garlic This antiviral and antibacterial allium can boost the immune system. Although it is best eaten raw, cooking does not greatly reduce its decongestant properties. Onions exhibit similar qualities.

Ginger This expectorant helps to fight colds and coughs.

Green tea The antiviral properties of this drink can help to reduce the likelihood of flu. It is rich in the antioxidant quercetin.

Turmeric This earthy spice is valued for its antibacterial and antifungal properties.

Recent studies indicate that turmeric may also reduce the risk of certain cancers.

Chillies These are an excellent source of vitamin C and are a good source of other antioxidants. They stimulate the body and are a powerful decongestant.

FOODS TO AVOID

Dairy products, caffeine, alcohol and processed foods all have a detrimental affect on the immune system, so should be consumed only in moderation.

Below: Oysters and crab are good sources of the immune-boosting mineral, zinc.

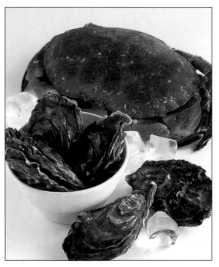

Shopping Essentials

• Fruit, especially citrus fruit, raspberries and strawberries, blackcurrants and bananas
• Vegetables, especially sweet potatoes, peppers, green leafy vegetables, carrots, avocados, watercress, onions and garlic
• Spices, especially chillies, ginger and turmeric
• Wholegrains, nuts and seeds
• Low-fat dairy produce and eggs
• Shellfish
• Beef, turkey and chicken
• Green tea

Looking After Your Digestive System

The condition of the digestive system often determines your general health. Everything you eat travels from the stomach to the intestines, where food is digested, nutrients absorbed and waste eliminated via the bowels. To break down food, we need "friendly" bacteria in the gut as well as digestive enzymes, which are produced by the stomach and small intestine. If these are out of balance due to poor diet, stress, antibiotics, food intolerances or toxin overload, food remains semi-digested. This is when conditions such as constipation, nausea, flatulence and indigestion can arise.

KEY PROTECTIVE FOODS FOR CONSTIPATION

Constipation is a common problem but if you eat correctly, drink plenty of water and take some exercise, symptoms can often be alleviated naturally, which is much better than resorting to laxatives.

Fresh fruit These stimulate the digestive system and are a good source of soluble fibre. A lack of fibre in the diet is the most common cause of constipation. You can also boost your intake by eating brown rice, wholegrain bread and pasta, dried fruit and fresh vegetables.

Live natural yogurt This can improve the condition of the gut and treat gastro-intestinal disorders. Live yogurt contains active beneficial bacteria, which can balance the intestinal microflora and promote good digestion, boost the immune system and increase resistance to infection. The symptoms of constipation, diarrhoea and IBS (irritable bowel syndrome) can all be relieved by eating live yogurt.

KEY PROTECTIVE FOODS FOR INDIGESTION

A number of factors can be responsible for indigestion, including stress and the consumption of fatty or spicy foods.

Below: Natural live yogurt provides a good source of beneficial bacteria to the gut.

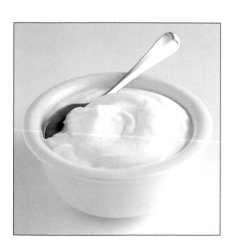

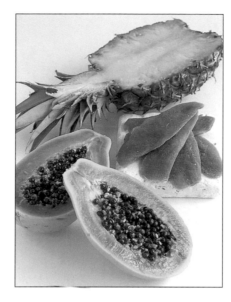

Above: Papaya, pineapple and mango contain an enzyme that helps in the digestion of meat.

Bananas Scientists have found that bananas may help to prevent and treat acid indigestion and also ulcers.

Pineapple and papaya Both these fruits can aid the digestion of protein found in meat. They contain enzymes – bromelain and papain respectively – which are natural meat tenderizers.

Ginger and peppermint These ingredients can help to soothe stomach cramps.

KEY PROTECTIVE FOODS FOR IRRITABLE BOWEL SYNDROME (IBS)

This painful condition is characterized by bloating, constipation, diarrhoea and cramps. It has been found that insoluble fibre, such as wheat bran, can further exacerbate the symptoms.

Herbal teas Tisanes, such as camomile, can soothe and calm the digestive system.

Fruit and vegetables These should be eaten frequently, as they are a good source of soluble fibre.

Live natural yogurt This can also help by improving the condition of the gut.

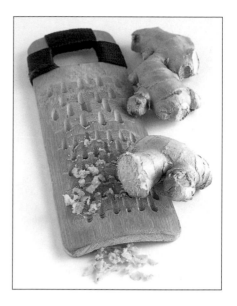

Above: Ginger has a calming effect on the digestive system.

KEY PROTECTIVE FOODS FOR FLATULENCE

Cutting down on pulses, cabbage and Brussels sprouts may help.

Spices Ginger, fennel, cinnamon and caraway are all said to have a calming influence on the digestive system.

Peppermint and basil A tisane made of these herbs may help to alleviate flatulence. Basil is also said to help relieve stomach cramps, nausea and constipation.

FOODS TO AVOID

Bran, spicy foods, alcohol and processed foods can all aggravate the gut.

Shopping Essentials
• Vegetables, except beans, cabbage and Brussels sprouts
• Fruit, especially bananas, pineapple and papaya
• Ginger, fennel, cinnamon and caraway seeds
• Live natural yogurt
• Herbal teas, especially camomile and peppermint

Eating to Ease Arthritis

Rheumatoid arthritis and osteoarthritis are the most common types of this disease. Rheumatoid arthritis is a complex condition, and its cause is still largely unknown. This inflammatory condition affects the joints and is thought to be related to a malfunctioning immune system. It can strike at any age. Osteoarthritis is a degenerative condition of the joints which occurs most commonly with age, and also tends to affect those who are overweight. There is no special diet for the treatment of osteoarthritis and experts question whether what you eat can prevent or relieve the painful symptoms. However, several recent studies suggest that antioxidants and fish oils may help.

Certain foods may bring relief to arthritis sufferers, but others can exacerbate the symptoms. If this happens, an allergy may be implicated, in which case consult an expert who may recommend an exclusion diet, followed by a tailor-made diet plan.

KEY FOODS

Vegetables and fruit Green leafy vegetables, carrots, broccoli, sweet potatoes, avocados, apricots, apples, bananas and mangoes will boost your intake of antioxidant nutrients such as vitamins C and E, betacarotene and selenium. These nutrients may protect cartilage from being destroyed by free radicals as well as helping to promote the growth of new cartilage. Asparagus has anti-inflammatory properties and soothes the pain and swelling of the joints.

Onions and kelp These contain quercetin, which is an anti-inflammatory agent.

Oily fish Salmon, tuna, mackerel, sardines and herrings have been shown to offer relief to sufferers of rheumatoid arthritis and may help those with osteoarthritis. It is recommended that oily fish be eaten about three times a week. Fish oils are rich in omega-3 fatty acids, which can help to reduce inflammation. For vegetarians, soya beans, tofu, linseeds, wheatgerm, walnuts and rapeseed oil are good alternative sources of omega-3 fatty acids. A meat-free diet is often recommended.

Spices Turmeric and fresh root ginger have anti-inflammatory properties.

New Zealand green-lipped mussels These molluscs are believed to reduce inflammation, although their therapeutic effect is yet to be proven.

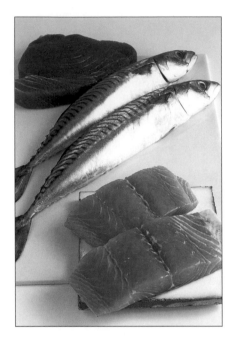

Above: Oily fish, such as tuna, mackerel and salmon, may relieve the symptoms of rheumatoid arthritis and osteoarthritis.

FOODS TO AVOID

It may help to cut down on or eliminate saturated fats and acidic foods, such as citrus fruit. Also avoid caffeine, red meat, sugar, alcohol, wheat, peppers, aubergines, tomatoes and potatoes.

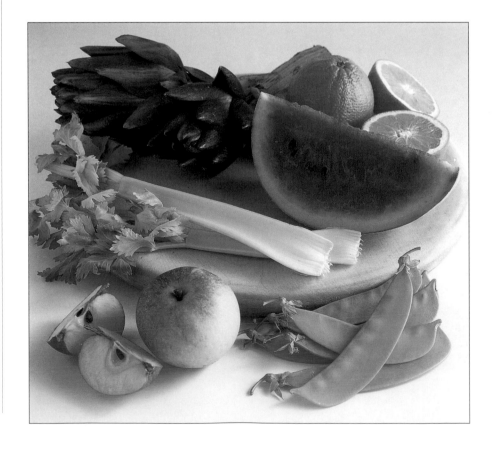

Below: Fresh fruit and vegetables are rich in antioxidant nutrients, which may help to protect cartilage from free radical damage.

Shopping Essentials

• Vegetables, especially green leafy vegetables, carrots, broccoli, avocados, asparagus, sweet potatoes and onions
• Fruit, especially apricots, apples, bananas and mangoes
• Oily fish
• Fish oils, rapeseed oil
• Kelp
• Tofu, soya beans
• Linseeds, wheatgerm, walnuts
• Turmeric and fresh root ginger

Healthy Skin, Hair and Nails

The condition of your skin, hair and nails is a reflection of your general health, which can be hindered by poor diet, pollution, stress, illness and lack of sleep. Plenty of fresh air, regular exercise, a healthy diet and at least eight glasses of water a day are the key to a glowing complexion, glossy hair and strong nails. However, genetic make-up also affects the skin, and parents can pass on the tendency to develop acne and eczema to their offspring.

KEY PROTECTIVE FOODS FOR THE SKIN

The skin is the largest organ in the body and is extremely vulnerable to the effects of modern living.

Fresh vegetables Carrots, spinach, sweet potatoes, broccoli, and apricots too, all provide betacarotene, an antioxidant. A deficiency can cause dry, itchy skin.

Fruit and nuts Citrus fruit, kiwi fruit, strawberries and other berries, avocados, vegetable oils, wholegrains, nuts, seeds, and some seafood all provide the antioxidant vitamins C and E, selenium and zinc, which help to transport nutrients to the skin and maintain collagen and elastin levels. Zinc-rich foods can improve skin conditions, such as eczema and psoriasis.

Apples and artichokes Apples are rich in pectin, which helps to cleanse the liver, thus aiding detoxification of the skin. Artichokes are also good liver cleansers, along with asparagus and beetroot. The latter is best eaten raw.

Fish, meat and eggs Fish, shellfish, wholegrains, meat and eggs provide B vitamins, which promote a glowing complexion and combat dryness.

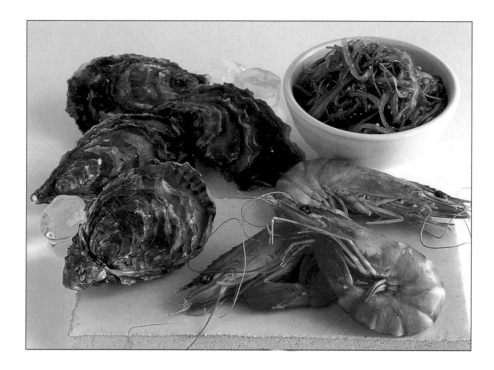

Above: Both shellfish and seaweed are rich in zinc, which is known to improve the condition of skin and nails.

Oily fish Essential fatty acids provided by mackerel, salmon, tuna, sardines and herrings, along with vegetable oils, nuts and seeds, can soften and hydrate the skin.

KEY PROTECTIVE FOODS FOR HAIR

Like the skin, your hair reflects your general state of health, and can be improved by a healthy diet and lifestyle.

Seaweed In Japan, a diet rich in seaweed is believed to give lustrous hair, probably owing to its high mineral content.

Meat and eggs Red meat, liver, fortified breakfast cereals, pulses and green leafy vegetables are also good sources of a wide range of minerals.

Dairy produce, nuts and pulses A good balance of protein foods including dairy produce, nuts and pulses, helps to keep your hair in good condition.

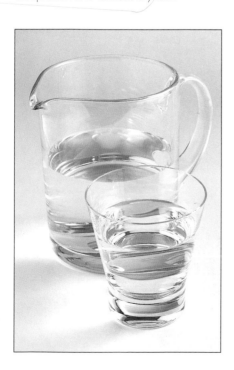

Left: Drinking eight glasses of water a day helps to keep skin, hair and nails healthy.

KEY FOODS FOR NAILS

Nails also respond favourably to a healthy diet, plenty of water and regular exercise. Certain minerals, including zinc, calcium and iron, keep them in good condition.

Green leafy vegetables These are recommended for healthy nail growth.

Nuts and seeds Good sources of calcium, these are easily included in the diet.

Dairy products and canned fish These are good sources of calcium.

Shopping Essentials

- Organic vegetables, especially sweet potatoes, carrots, spinach, broccoli, artichokes, asparagus and beetroot
- Organic fruit, especially apricots, citrus, kiwi fruit, berries and apples
- Fresh and canned fish, especially oily fish, and shellfish
- Wholegrains, nuts, seeds and pulses
- Vegetable oil
- Fortified breakfast cereals
- Poultry and meat, especially red meat and liver
- Eggs and low-fat dairy produce

Women's Health

Women have their own particular concerns and problems when it comes to their health. Diet, combined with regular exercise and a healthy lifestyle, plays a crucial role in helping to balance hormonal levels that can affect women's health.

KEY PROTECTIVE FOODS FOR PRE-MENSTRUAL SYNDROME (PMS)

This is the name given to the physical and mental changes that can occur 2–14 days before menstruation. The symptoms, which include bloating, constipation, diarrhoea, mood swings and food cravings, can be alleviated by manipulating the diet. Wheatgerm, wholegrains, bananas, oily fish, and poultry are good sources of vitamin B_6, which is especially helpful in combatting water retention and breast tenderness and can also aid the absorption of magnesium. A lack of magnesium can increase the likelihood of PMS, particularly the symptoms of mood swings and cravings.

Dried apricots, liver, red meat, pulses, eggs, green leafy vegetables, fortified breakfast cereals, seeds and wholegrains These foods are rich in iron and help to avert the symptoms of iron deficiency, such as anaemia and fatigue.

Citrus fruits, kiwi fruits and blackcurrants It is important to eat plenty of foods rich in vitamin C, which is necessary for the uptake of iron into the bloodstream. This is particularly important for women who have heavy or prolonged periods.

Below: Oily fish, dried apricots and spinach can help to alleviate the symptoms of pre-menstrual syndrome.

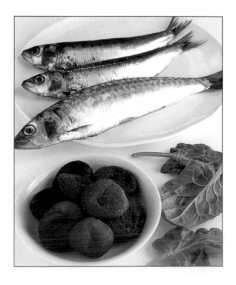

Oily fish, sunflower oil, rapeseed oil, nuts and seeds These contain essential fatty acids, which can to help reduce breast pain.
Vegetable oils, nuts, avocados, eggs and wheatgerm These contain Vitamin E, which can also help to relieve breast pain.
Raspberries These soft fruits are said to help alleviate stomach cramps.

CYSTITIS

Affecting over twice as many women as men, cystitis can cause much discomfort.
Cranberry juice This fruit juice provides relief for several urinary tract disorders. Originally, it was thought to increase the acidity of urine which destroyed bacteria causing the infection. However, new research shows that compounds in the berries' natural sugar bind to the bacteria, which are then removed with the urine.
Water As with any urinary tract infection, it is important to drink plenty of water.

PREGNANCY

The health of a mother affects the health of her child both at birth and through to his or her adulthood. Expectant mothers and women planning to become pregnant should follow the basic guidelines of a healthy diet and should also increase intake of certain nutrients.

Dark green vegetables, soya beans, eggs, yeast extract, fortified breakfast cereals and nuts These are rich in folic acid, which can help to reduce the risk of spina bifida.
Soya products, dairy products, meat, yeast extract and eggs These provide vitamin B_{12}, which works alongside folic acid to form red blood cells.
Dark green leafy vegetables and dairy products These offer a good supply of calcium, which is needed to ensure healthy bone development in the foetus.
Eggs, dried apricots, meat, fortified breakfast cereals, pulses, green leafy vegetables and wholegrains These foods are rich in iron, which is needed to create haemoglobin and prevent anaemia.

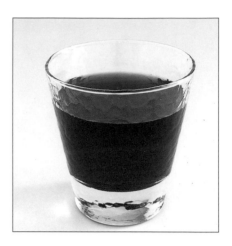

Above: Cranberry juice is an effective and palatable way of treating cystitis.

Fresh root ginger, wheatgerm, oily fish, bananas, wholegrains and poultry These foods can help relieve morning sickness.

MENOPAUSE

Many women suffer from the side effects, of menopause, which include depression, insomnia and anxiety, together with hot flushes and night sweats.

There has been much interest in the possible role of phytoestrogens in the relief of menopausal symptoms, such as hot flushes and vaginitis (inflammation of the vagina). Hormone replacement therapy (HRT) can alleviate these but foods containing phytoestrogens, such as soya beans, tofu, soya milk and linseeds, are said to be good natural alternatives.
Soya products These may help to maintain bone density and are believed to reduce the risk of breast cancer.
Sweet potatoes These contain natural progesterone and may help menopausal symptoms and hormone imbalance.
Low-fat dairy products, nuts, seeds, green leafy vegetables, canned fish, pulses, soya products, seaweed and bread These calcium-rich foods can help to slow down bone density loss during menopause, thus reducing the risk of osteoporosis. Foods rich in vitamin D, zinc and magnesium are also important.

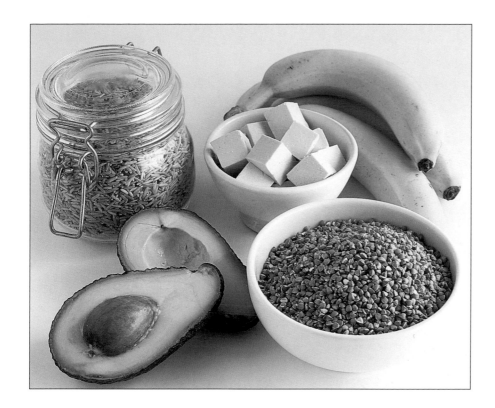

Above: Wholegrains, avocados, bananas and tofu are all believed to be beneficial to women's health.

Osteoporosis

This condition occurs when bone mass diminishes. Bones become fragile and susceptible to fracture. It is most common among post-menopausal women, although it can affect people of all ages and both sexes. Certain dietary measures can reduce the risk of osteoporosis.

Fruit and vegetables These may be important for good bone health and

Below: Dairy products provide calcium, which can help to reduce the risk of osteoporosis.

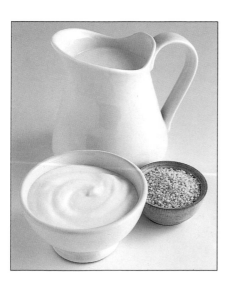

the prevention of osteoporosis. Unlike some foods that increase acidity in the body and encourage minerals to be drawn out of the bones to neutralize the acid, fruit and vegetables create a more alkaline environment, and so help to prevent the loss of bone mineral density.

Low-fat dairy products, sardines, green leafy vegetables, almonds, Brazil nuts and figs These foods are rich in calcium, the main constituent of bone. Eating calcium-rich foods, particularly in childhood and adolescence, can help to reduce the risk of osteoporosis in later life.

Nuts, seeds, soya products and whole-grain cereals These are good sources of magnesium, which works in tandem with calcium and is important for bone health.

Oily fish, green leafy vegetables, margarine and fortified breakfast cereals These provide vitamin D, which is also obtained by the action of sunlight on skin. It is needed for the assimilation of calcium.

Soya This is not only a rich source of isoflavones (phytoestrogens), but it is also a good source of calcium. There is a much lower incidence of osteoporosis among Japanese women, which has been linked to their higher intake of soya products.

Foods to Avoid

Keep intake of fatty and sugary foods to a minimum. Also restrict the amount of tea, coffee and alcohol you drink, as these can diminish absorption of vital nutrients.

Shopping Essentials

For Pre-menstrual Syndrome
• Green leafy vegetables and avocados
• Wholegrains, pulses, wheatgerm, seeds and nuts
• Oily fish
• Fruit, especially bananas, raspberries and dried apricots
• Red meat, liver, poultry
• Eggs
• Fortified breakfast cereals
• Sunflower oil and rapeseed oil

For Menopause
• Green leafy vegetables and sweet potatoes
• Soya beans, soya milk and tofu
• Seaweed
• Nuts and seeds, especially linseeds
• Pulses
• Low-fat dairy products
• Canned fish
• Bread

For Pregnancy
• Dark green vegetables
• Fruit, especially bananas
• Soya beans
• Yeast extract
• Dairy products and eggs
• Lean meat
• Oily fish and poultry
• Wholegrains, pulses, wheatgerm and nuts
• Fortified breakfast cereals
• Fresh root ginger

For Osteoporosis
• Fruit and vegetables, especially figs and green leafy vegetables
• Low-fat dairy products
• Margarine
• Brazil nuts and seeds
• Soya products
• Wholegrain cereals
• Oily fish
• Fortified breakfast cereals

Protecting Against Cancer

A recent report by the World Cancer Research Fund claims that up to 40 per cent of cancers could be prevented by a healthy diet and lifestyle. Scientific evidence supports the argument that certain foods, when eaten as part of a healthy balanced diet, may help to reduce the risk of cancer and may also play a role in supporting medical treatment.

KEY PROTECTIVE FOODS

A diet rich in fruit and vegetables is thought to be the key to reducing the risk of cancer, owing to their antioxidant vitamins and minerals, phytochemicals and fibre content.

Carrots, sweet potatoes and broccoli These vegetables contain carotenoids, which may help to fight lung cancer.

Citrus fruit These fruits provide vitamin C, which is believed to protect against cancer of the oesophagus and stomach.

Tomatoes These vegetables contain lycopene, which is a powerful antioxidant.

Wholegrains, pulses and potatoes These foods provide rich amounts of fibre, which may help to reduce the risk of cancer of the large intestine, prostate and breast.

Garlic, onions, leeks and chives These alliums, especially when eaten raw, may protect against cancers of the colon, breast and liver.

Below: Yam, oriental mushrooms, carrots, beetroot and broccoli all contain rich supplies of cancer-fighting nutrients.

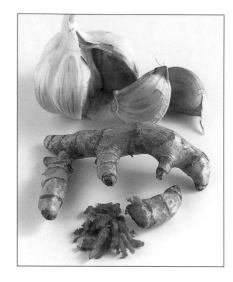

Above: Garlic and turmeric are reputed to reduce the risk of certain cancers.

Soya beans and soya products These are rich in isoflavones, which are believed to reduce the risk of hormone-dependent cancers, such as breast and prostate.

Green tea This tea not only contains less caffeine than black tea, but may protect against certain cancers, including those that affect the colon, pancreas and rectum.

Fish Research has shown that a diet rich in fish, especially oily fish, can reduce the risk of cancer of the digestive tract. The essential fatty acids found in oily fish and many cooking oils are said to have be anti-inflammatory and inhibit the growth of cancer cells.

FOODS TO AVOID

Fat, especially saturated fat, has been linked to an increased risk of lung, breast, prostate and bowel cancer. Red meat has been linked with an increased risk of cancers of the colon and rectum. Smoked foods, such as smoked salmon, bacon and kippers, as well as barbecued and chargrilled food, may increase the risk of cancer. Salt, taken in excessive amounts, may increase the risk of stomach cancer.

Below: Green tea is believed to fight against cancer of the colon, pancreas and rectum.

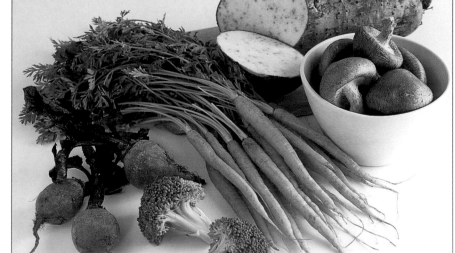

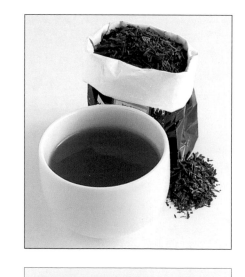

Shopping Essentials
- Fruit, especially citrus fruit
- Vegetables, especially potatoes, sweet potatoes, carrots, broccoli, tomatoes and garlic, onions and other members of the onion family
- Fish, especially oily fish
- Soya products
- Green tea

Eating with Diabetes

Diabetes mellitus is becoming increasingly common. It is caused by a lack of the hormone insulin, which is required to regulate blood sugar levels. There are two types of diabetes: insulin-dependent and non-insulin-dependent. People who are insulin dependent do not produce any insulin themselves and require regular injections of insulin, supported by a healthy diet and lifestyle. Those people who are non-insulin-dependent produce small amounts of insulin but not enough. This type is more common among older people and those who are overweight. Non-insulin-dependent diabetes can be controlled through diet alone but may sometimes also require medication.

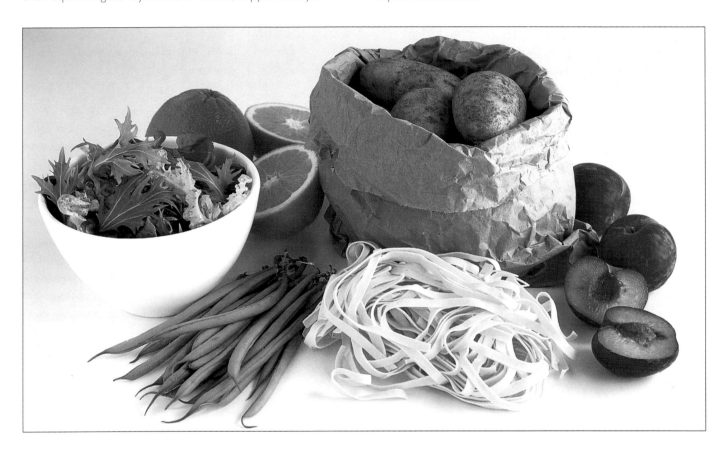

KEY PROTECTIVE FOODS

Wholegrain cereals, wholemeal bread and pasta, brown rice and potatoes with their skins on It is important to maintain and stabilize blood sugar levels by eating high-fibre, starchy foods, which provide a steady release of sugar and energy into the system. Sweet foods can be eaten occasionally but eat them after a starchy meal to keep blood sugar levels steady.

Vegetables These provide valuable amounts of fibre, vitamins and minerals.

Fruit Although fruit does contain a type of sugar called fructose, its high fibre content helps to stabilize the release of the sugar into the bloodstream. Pears, apples and oranges all provide a good balance of sugar and fibre.

FOODS TO AVOID

Avoid sugary foods and drinks. Diabetics have an increased risk of heart disease and should, therefore, keep fat intake, particularly of saturated fat, to a minimum. Opt instead for low-fat sources of protein, such as lean meat, poultry without the skin, fish, pulses, soya and low-fat dairy produce. Eggs may be eaten occasionally.

Shopping Essentials

• Fresh vegetables of all types, including potatoes

• Fruit, particularly pears, apples and oranges

• Wholegrain cereals, wholemeal bread and wholemeal pasta

• Brown rice, pulses

• Lean meat and poultry

• Fish

• Soya products

• Low-fat dairy products

Above: Unrefined starchy foods, as well as fresh fruit and vegetables, help to keep blood-sugar levels stable.

Below: It is important to keep intake of high-sugar foods such as cakes, biscuits and sugary fizzy drinks, to a minimum.

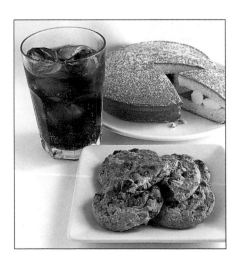

Banana and Strawberry Smoothie

FULL OF ENERGY-GIVING OATS and fruits, this tasty drink makes a brilliant breakfast.

INGREDIENTS
2 bananas, quartered
250g/9oz/2 cups strawberries
30ml/2 tbsp oatmeal
500g/1¼lb/2½ cups natural
    live yogurt
Serves 2

COOK'S TIP

Prepare fruit drinks just before serving to gain maximum benefit from the nutrients.

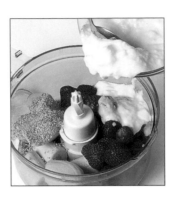

Place the bananas, strawberries, oatmeal and yogurt in a food processor or blender and process for a few minutes until combined and creamy. Pour into tall glasses and serve.

Citrus Shake

PACKED WITH VITAMIN C, this refreshing juice is a great way to start the day.

INGREDIENTS
1 pineapple
6 oranges, peeled and chopped
juice of 1 lemon
1 pink grapefruit, peeled and
    chopped
Serves 4

1 To prepare the pineapple, cut the bottom and the spiky top off the fruit. Stand the pineapple upright and cut off the skin, removing all the spikes and as little of the flesh as possible. Lay the pineapple on its side and cut into bite-size chunks.

2 Place the pineapple, oranges, lemon juice and grapefruit in a food processor or blender and process for a few minutes until combined.

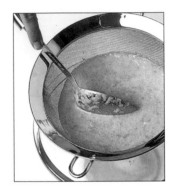

3 Press the fruit juice through a sieve to remove any pith or membranes. Serve chilled.

Cranberry and Apple Juice

THIS GINGER-FLAVOURED, CLEANSING JUICE offers a fine balance of sweet and sour tastes.

INGREDIENTS
4 eating apples
600ml/1 pint/2½ cups
    cranberry juice
2.5cm/1in piece fresh root
    ginger, peeled and sliced
Serves 4

HEALTH BENEFITS

Brightly coloured fruits, such as cranberries, contain valuable amounts of antioxidant vitamins, which are believed to have cancer-fighting properties.

1 Peel the apples, if you wish, then core and chop.

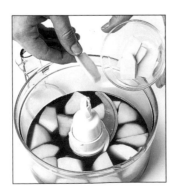

2 Pour the cranberry juice into a food processor or blender. Add the chopped apples and sliced ginger and process for a few minutes until combined and fairly smooth. Serve chilled.

Zingy Vegetable Juice

GINGER PACKS A POWERFUL punch and certainly gets you going in the morning, even if you're feeling groggy.

INGREDIENTS
1 cooked beetroot in natural
    juice, sliced
1 large carrot, sliced
4cm/1½in piece fresh root
    ginger, peeled and finely grated
2 apples, peeled, if liked,
    chopped and cored
150g/5oz/1¼ cups seedless
    white grapes
300ml/½ pint/1¼ cups fresh
    orange juice
Serves 2

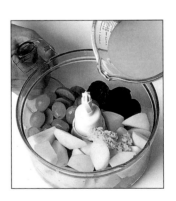

1 Place the beetroot, carrot, ginger, apples, grapes and orange juice in a food processor or blender and process for a few minutes until combined and fairly smooth. Serve immediately or chill until ready to serve.

Right: Clockwise from top right, Cranberry and Apple Juice, Citrus Shake, Banana and Strawberry Smoothie, Zingy Vegetable Juice.

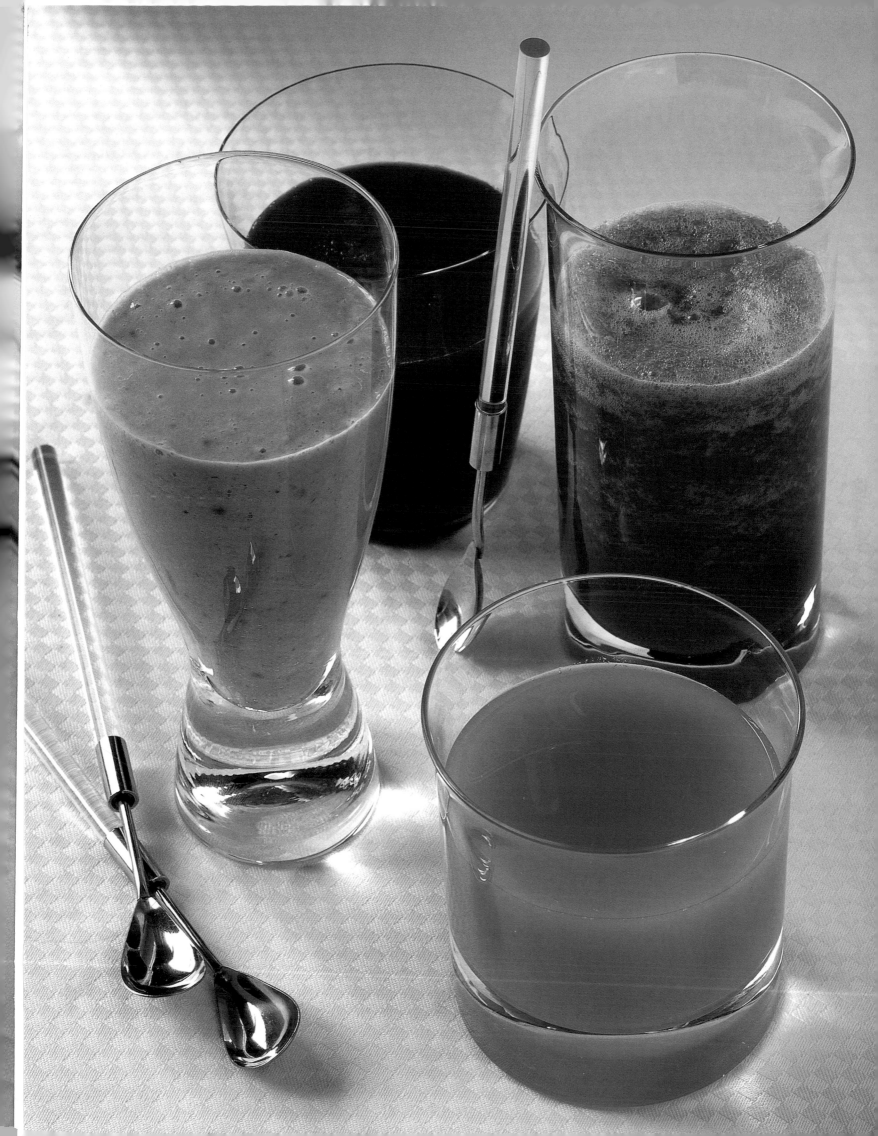

Kedgeree

THIS SPICY LENTIL AND RICE dish is a delicious variation of the original Indian version of kedgeree, *kitchiri*. You can serve it as it is, or topped with quartered hard-boiled eggs if you'd like to add more protein. It is also delicious served on grilled, large field mushrooms.

INGREDIENTS

50g/2oz/¼ cup dried red lentils, rinsed
1 bay leaf
225g/8oz/1 cup basmati rice, rinsed
4 cloves
50g/2oz/4 tbsp butter
5ml/1 tsp curry powder
2.5ml/½ tsp mild chilli powder
30ml/2 tbsp chopped flat leaf parsley
salt and freshly ground black pepper
4 hard-boiled eggs, quartered, to serve
*   (optional)*
Serves 4

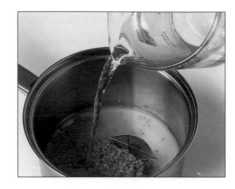

1 Put the lentils in a saucepan, add the bay leaf and cover with cold water. Bring to the boil, skim off any foam, then reduce the heat. Cover and simmer for 25–30 minutes, until tender. Drain, then discard the bay leaf.

2 Meanwhile, place the rice in a saucepan and cover with 475ml/ 16fl oz/2 cups boiling water. Add the cloves and a generous pinch of salt. Cook, covered, for 10–15 minutes, until all the water is absorbed and the rice is tender. Discard the cloves.

3 Melt the butter over a gentle heat in a large frying pan, then add the curry and chilli powders and cook for 1 minute.

4 Stir in the lentils and rice and mix well until they are coated in the spiced butter. Season and cook for 1–2 minutes until heated through. Stir in the parsley and serve with the hard-boiled eggs, if using.

HEALTH BENEFITS

• Lentils are especially good for the heart, because of their ability to lower cholesterol levels in the body. They also contain compounds that inhibit cancer and can regulate blood sugar levels.
• Rice is a high-carbohydrate food that provides sustained amounts of energy, making it a perfect food to start the day. Rice can also help to ease diarrhoea and stomach upsets.

Griddled Tomatoes on Soda Bread

START YOUR DAY WITH THESE DELICIOUS tomatoes served on soda bread to give your body a generous boost of health-giving phytochemicals and plenty of long-term energy.

INGREDIENTS

olive oil, for brushing and drizzling
6 tomatoes, thickly sliced
4 thick slices soda bread
balsamic vinegar, for drizzling
salt and freshly ground black pepper
shavings of Parmesan cheese, to serve
Serves 4

COOK'S TIP

Using a griddle pan reduces the amount of oil required for cooking the tomatoes and gives them a barbecued flavour.

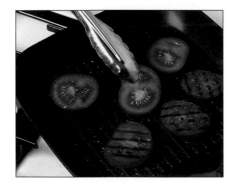

1 Brush a griddle pan with olive oil and heat. Add the tomato slices and cook for about 4 minutes, turning once, until softened and slightly blackened. Alternatively, heat a grill to high and line the rack with foil. Grill the tomato slices for 4–6 minutes, turning once, until softened.

2 Meanwhile, lightly toast the soda bread. Place the tomatoes on top of the toast and drizzle each portion with a little olive oil and vinegar. Season to taste and serve immediately with thin shavings of Parmesan.

HEALTH BENEFITS

Numerous studies have shown that tomatoes are effective in preventing many forms of cancer, including lung, stomach and prostate cancer. This is probably explained by their antioxidant content, notably betacarotene and vitamins C and E. Antioxidants are also believed to prevent appendicitis.

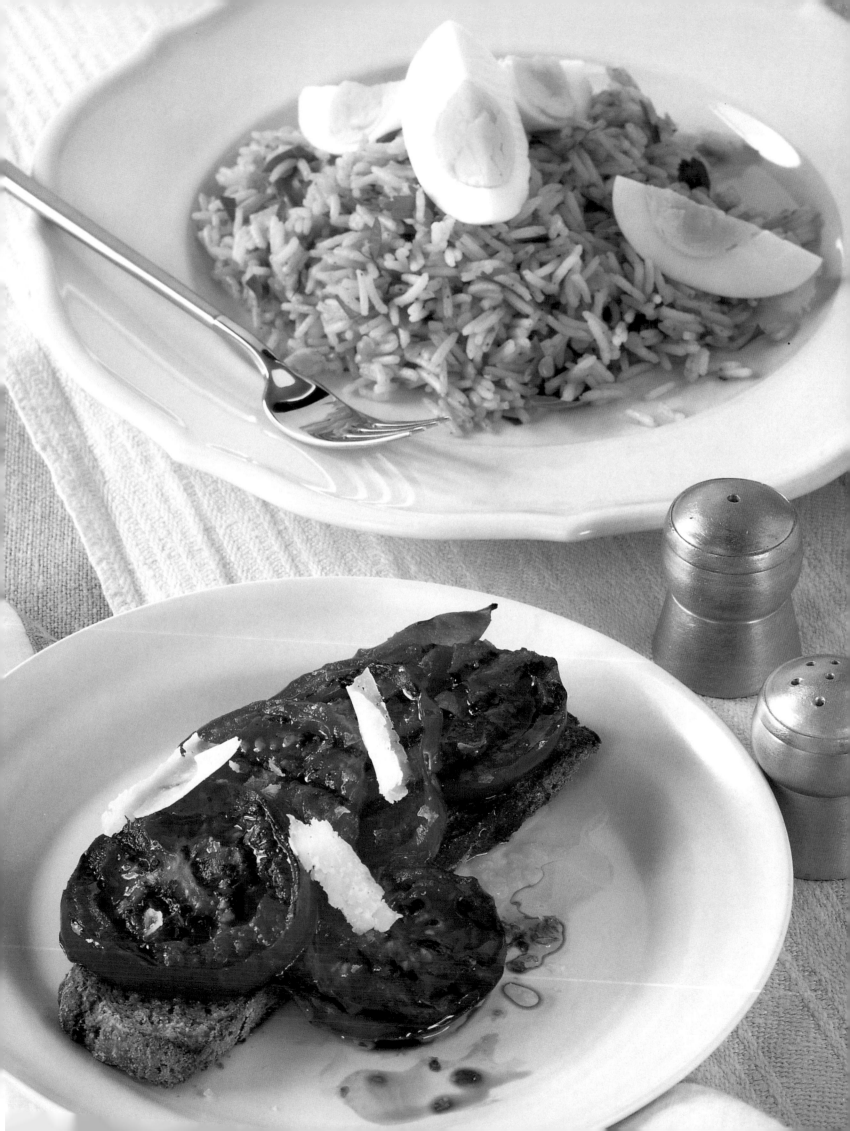

Porridge with Date Purée and Pistachio Nuts

FULL OF VALUABLE FIBRE AND nutrients, dates give a natural sweet flavour to this warming winter breakfast dish.

INGREDIENTS

250g/9oz/scant 2 cups fresh dates
225g/8oz/2 cups rolled oats
475ml/16fl oz/2 cups semi-skimmed milk
pinch of salt
50g/2oz/¹/2 cup shelled, unsalted pistachio
    nuts, roughly chopped
Serves 4

HEALTH BENEFITS

Oats have a reputation for being warming foods due to their fat and protein content, which is greater than that of most other grains. As well as providing energy and endurance, oats are one of the most nutritious cereals.

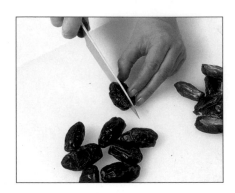

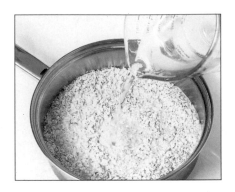

1 First make the date purée. Halve the dates and remove the stones and stems. Cover the dates with boiling water and leave to soak for about 30 minutes, until softened. Strain, reserving 90ml/6 tbsp of the soaking water.

2 Remove the skin from the dates and place them in a food processor with the reserved soaking water. Process to a smooth purée.

3 Place the oats in a saucepan with the milk, 300ml/¹/2 pint/1¹/4 cups water and salt. Bring to the boil, then reduce the heat and simmer for 4–5 minutes until cooked and creamy, stirring frequently.

4 Serve the porridge in warm serving bowls, topped with a spoonful of the date purée and sprinkled with chopped pistachio nuts.

Apricot and Ginger Compote

FRESH GINGER ADDS WARMTH to this stimulating breakfast dish and complements the flavour of the plump, juicy apricots.

INGREDIENTS

350g/12oz/1¹/2 cups dried unsulphured
    apricots
4cm/1¹/2in piece fresh root ginger,
    finely chopped
200g/7oz/scant 1 cup natural live yogurt
    or low-fat fromage frais
Serves 4

COOK'S TIP

Fresh ginger freezes well. Peel the root and store it in a plastic bag in the freezer. You can grate it from frozen, then return the root to the freezer until the next time you need it for a recipe.

1 Cover the apricots with boiling water, then leave to soak overnight.

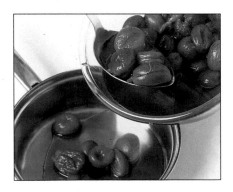

2 Place the apricots and their soaking water in a saucepan, add the ginger and bring to the boil. Reduce the heat and simmer for 10 minutes until the fruit is soft and plump and the water becomes syrupy. Strain the apricots, reserving the syrup, and discard the ginger.

3 Serve the apricots warm with the reserved syrup and a spoonful of yogurt or fromage frais.

HEALTH BENEFITS

• *In Chinese medicine, ginger is revered for its health-giving properties. It is said to aid digestion and can help treat colds and flu.*

• *Of all the dried fruits, apricots are the richest source of iron. They also provide calcium, phosphorus and vitamins A and C.*

• *Live yogurt can relieve gastrointestinal disorders by replacing valuable bacteria in the gut. The lactic acids, which yogurt contains, can help to regulate bowel function and they have bacterial properties that can prevent infection. Yogurt also boosts our immune system.*

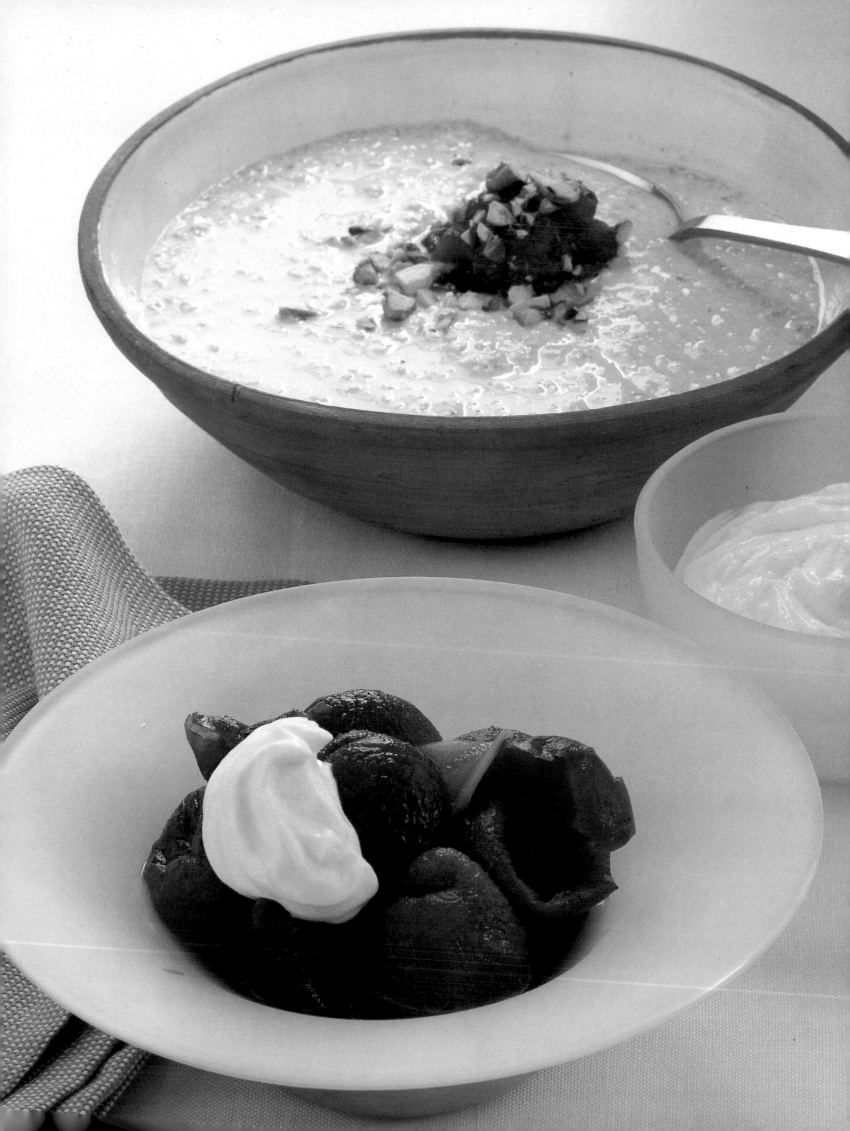

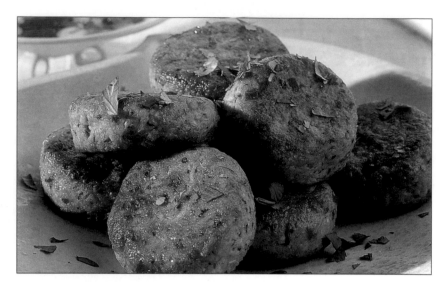

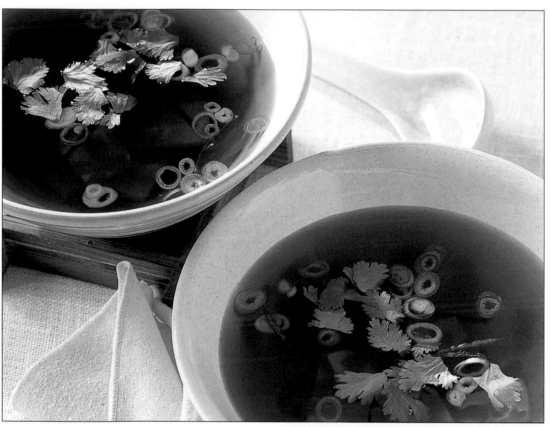

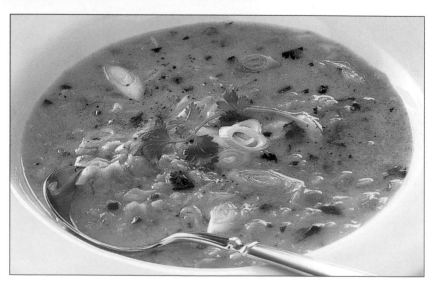

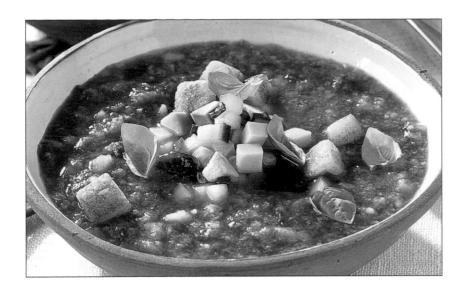

SOUPS AND LIGHT MEALS

Warming soup is the perfect health food. It is a great way of serving

vegetables, and many children who scorn salads will happily accept

a puréed vegetable soup. Try Roasted Root Vegetable Soup, and

Gazpacho with Avocado Salsa. The selection of light meals is equally

enticing and offers such temptations as Cannellini Bean and Rosemary

Bruschetta, and Thai Tempeh Cakes with Sweet Dipping Sauce.

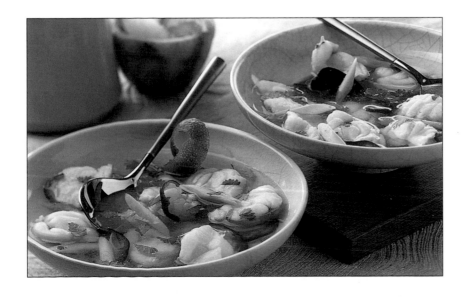

Gazpacho with Avocado Salsa

TOMATOES, CUCUMBERS AND peppers form the basis of this classic, chilled soup and provide a powerhouse of nutrients. Add a spoonful of chunky, fresh avocado salsa to give your hair and skin an extra health boost.

INGREDIENTS

2 slices day-old bread
1kg/2¼lb tomatoes
1 cucumber
1 red pepper, seeded and chopped
1 green chilli, seeded and chopped
2 garlic cloves, chopped
30ml/2 tbsp extra virgin olive oil
juice of 1 lime and 1 lemon
a few drops Tabasco sauce
salt and freshly ground black pepper
a handful of basil leaves, to garnish
8 ice cubes, to serve

For the croûtons
2 slices day-old bread, crusts removed
1 garlic clove, halved
15ml/1 tbsp olive oil

For the avocado salsa
1 ripe avocado
5ml/1 tsp lemon juice
2.5cm/1in piece cucumber, diced
½ red chilli, finely chopped
Serves 4

1 Soak the bread in 150ml/¼ pint/ ⅔ cup of water for 5 minutes.

2 Meanwhile, place the tomatoes in a bowl and cover with boiling water. Leave for 30 seconds, then peel, seed and chop the flesh.

HEALTH BENEFITS

The powerful combination of fresh raw vegetables, garlic, lemon and lime juice, olive oil and chilli boosts the immune system and the circulation, and helps to cleanse the body.

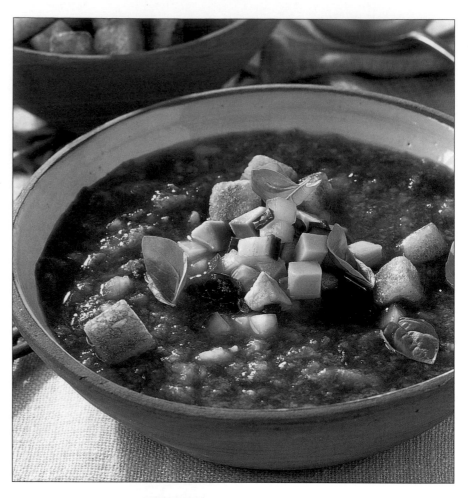

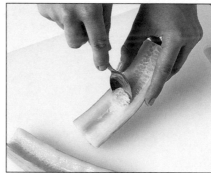

3 Thinly peel the cucumber, then cut it in half lengthways and scoop out the seeds with a teaspoon. Discard the seeds and chop the flesh.

4 Place the bread, tomatoes, cucumber, red pepper, chilli, garlic, olive oil, citrus juices and Tabasco in a food processor or blender with 450ml/¾ pint/scant 2 cups chilled water and blend until well combined but still chunky. Season to taste and chill for 2–3 hours.

5 To make the croûtons, rub the slices of bread with the garlic clove. Cut the bread into cubes and place in a plastic bag with the olive oil. Seal the bag and shake until the bread cubes are coated with the oil. Heat a large non-stick frying pan and fry the croûtons over a medium heat until crisp and golden.

6 Just before serving, make the avocado salsa. Halve the avocado, remove the stone, then peel and dice. Toss the avocado in the lemon juice to prevent it browning, then mix with the cucumber and chilli.

7 Ladle the soup into bowls, add the ice cubes, and top with a spoonful of avocado salsa. Garnish with the basil and hand round the croûtons separately.

Japanese-style Noodle Soup

THIS DELICATE, FRAGRANT SOUP is flavoured with just a hint of chilli and will make the perfect light lunch. It will keep you going through the day with its combination of noodles and fresh vegetables.

INGREDIENTS

45ml/3 tbsp mugi miso
200g/7oz/scant 2 cups udon noodles,
    soba noodles or Chinese noodles
30ml/2 tbsp sake or dry sherry
15ml/1 tbsp rice or wine vinegar
45ml/3 tbsp Japanese soy sauce
115g/4oz asparagus tips or mangetouts,
    thinly sliced diagonally
50g/2oz/scant 1 cup shiitake mushrooms,
    stalks removed and thinly sliced
1 carrot, sliced into julienne strips
3 spring onions, thinly sliced diagonally
salt and freshly ground black pepper
5ml/1 tsp dried chilli flakes, to serve
Serves 4

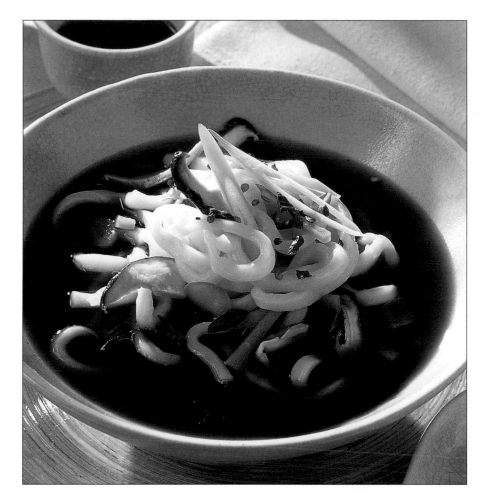

1 Bring 1 litre/1¾ pints/4 cups water to the boil in a saucepan. Pour 150ml/¼ pint/⅔ cup of the boiling water over the miso and stir until dissolved, then set aside.

2 Meanwhile, bring another large pan of lightly salted water to the boil, add the noodles and cook according to the packet instructions until just tender.

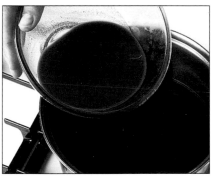

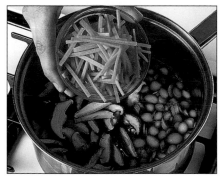

4 Add the sake or sherry, rice or wine vinegar and soy sauce to the pan of boiling water. Boil gently for 3 minutes or until the alcohol has evaporated, then reduce the heat and stir in the miso mixture.

5 Add the asparagus or mange-touts, mushrooms, carrot and spring onions, and simmer for about 2 minutes until the vegetables are just tender. Season to taste.

6 Divide the noodles among four warm bowls and pour the soup over the top. Serve immediately, sprinkled with the chilli flakes.

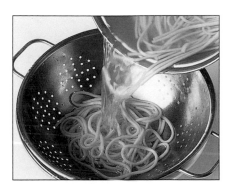

3 Drain the noodles in a colander. Rinse under cold running water, then drain again.

HEALTH BENEFITS

Miso shares many of the health qualities of soya. It has shown itself to be effective against stomach cancer, which no doubt stems from its antioxidant qualities.

Italian Pea and Basil Soup

NUTRIENT-RICH PEAS and therapeutic basil make the perfect combination.

INGREDIENTS
75ml/5 tbsp olive oil
2 large onions, chopped
1 celery stick, chopped
1 carrot, chopped
1 garlic clove, finely chopped
400g/14oz/3¹/₂ cups frozen petit pois
900ml/1¹/₂ pints/3³/₄ cups vegetable stock
25g/1oz/1 cup fresh basil leaves, roughly
    torn, plus extra to garnish
salt and freshly ground black pepper
freshly grated Parmesan cheese, to serve
Serves 4

VARIATION

Use mint or a mixture of parsley, mint and chives in place of the basil.

1 Heat the oil in a large saucepan and add the onions, celery, carrot and garlic. Cover the pan and cook over a low heat for 45 minutes or until the vegetables are soft, stirring occasionally to prevent the vegetables sticking.

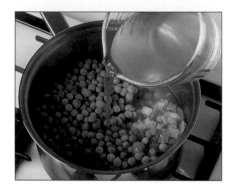

2 Add the peas and stock to the pan and bring to the boil. Reduce the heat, add the basil and seasoning, then simmer for 10 minutes.

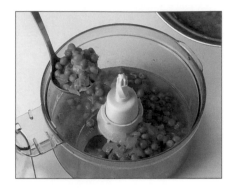

3 Spoon the soup into a food processor or blender and process until the soup is smooth. Ladle into warm bowls, sprinkle with grated Parmesan and garnish with basil.

HEALTH BENEFITS

As freezing usually takes place soon after picking, frozen peas may have a higher vitamin C content than fresh.

Spiced Red Lentil and Coconut Soup

HOT, SPICY AND RICHLY FLAVOURED, this substantial soup is almost a meal in itself. If you are really hungry, serve with chunks of warmed naan bread or thick slices of toast.

INGREDIENTS
30ml/2 tbsp sunflower oil
2 red onions, finely chopped
1 bird's eye chilli, seeded and finely sliced
2 garlic cloves, chopped
2.5cm/1in piece fresh lemon grass, outer
    layers removed and inside finely sliced
200g/7oz/scant 1 cup red lentils, rinsed
5ml/1 tsp ground coriander
5ml/1 tsp paprika
400ml/14fl oz/1²/₃ cups coconut milk
juice of 1 lime
3 spring onions, chopped
20g/³/₄oz/scant 1 cup fresh coriander,
    finely chopped
salt and freshly ground black pepper
Serves 4

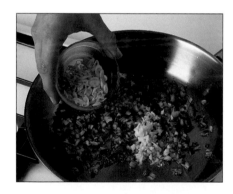

1 Heat the oil in a large pan and add the onions, chilli, garlic and lemon grass. Cook for 5 minutes or until the onions have softened but not browned, stirring occasionally.

HEALTH BENEFITS

Lentils provide a rich supply of minerals, including iron and calcium, as well as folic acid. The latter is recommended for pregnant women as it can lower the risk of spina bifida in the unborn child.

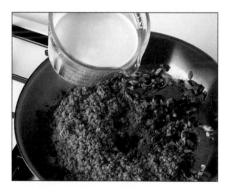

2 Add the lentils and spices. Pour in the coconut milk and 900ml/1¹/₂ pints/3³/₄ cups water, and stir. Bring to the boil, stir, then reduce the heat and simmer for 40–45 minutes or until the lentils are soft and mushy.

3 Pour in the lime juice and add the spring onions and fresh coriander, reserving a little of each for the garnish. Season, then ladle into bowls. Garnish with the reserved spring onions and coriander.

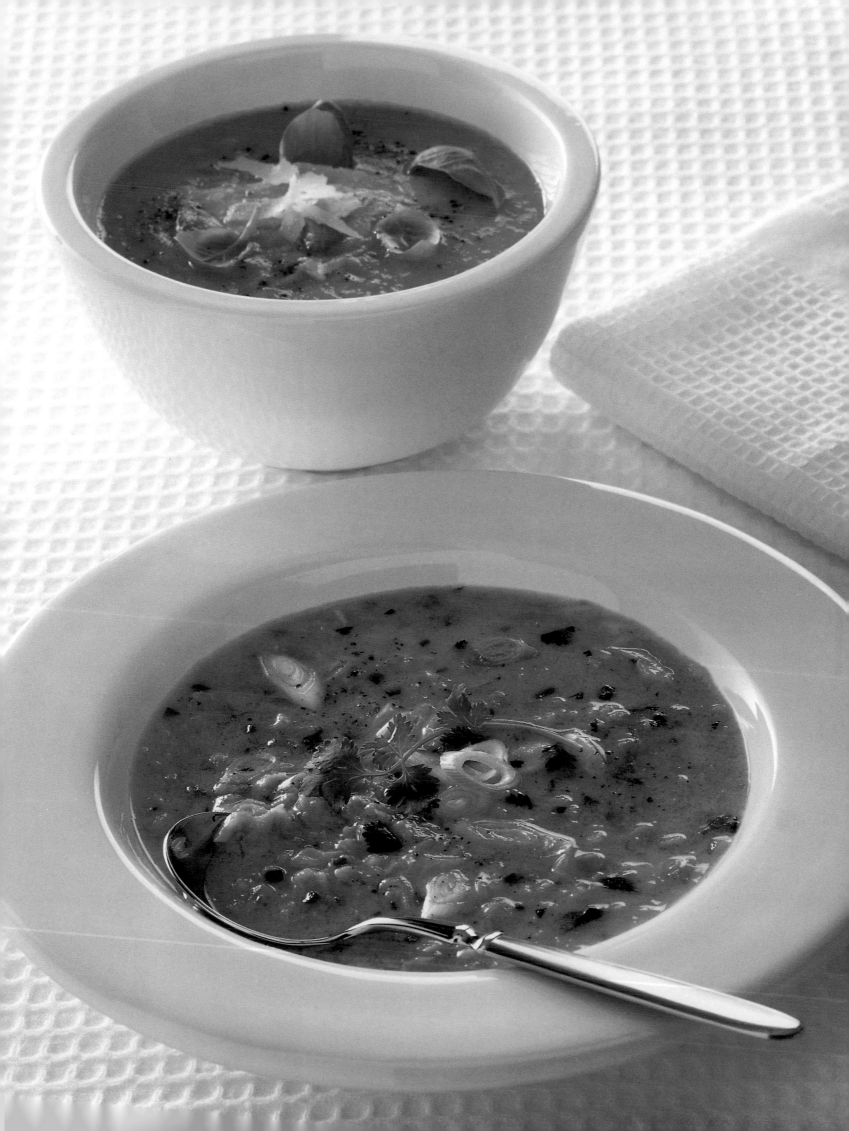

Hot-and-sour Soup

THIS LIGHT AND INVIGORATING soup originates from Thailand. It is best served at the beginning of a Thai meal to stimulate the appetite.

INGREDIENTS

2 carrots

900ml/1 1/2 pints/3 3/4 cups vegetable stock

2 Thai chillies, seeded and finely sliced

2 lemon grass stalks, outer leaves removed and each stalk cut into 3 pieces

4 kaffir lime leaves

2 garlic cloves, finely chopped

4 spring onions, finely sliced

5ml/1 tsp sugar

juice of 1 lime

45ml/3 tbsp chopped fresh coriander

salt

130g/4 1/2oz/1 cup Japanese tofu, sliced

Serves 4

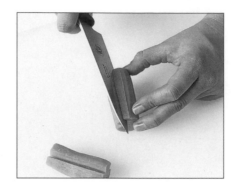

1 To make carrot flowers, cut each carrot in half crossways, then, using a sharp knife, cut four v-shaped channels lengthways. Slice the carrots into thin rounds and set aside.

COOK'S TIP

Kaffir lime leaves have a distinctive citrus flavour. The fresh leaves can be bought from Asian shops, and some supermarkets now sell them dried.

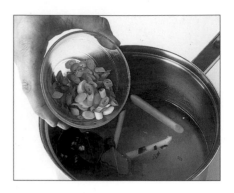

2 Pour the stock into a large saucepan. Reserve 2.5ml/1/2 tsp of the chillies and add the rest to the pan with the lemon grass, lime leaves, garlic and half the spring onions. Bring to the boil, then reduce the heat and simmer for 20 minutes. Strain the stock and discard the flavourings.

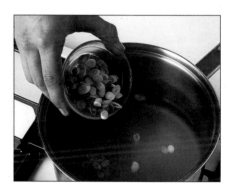

3 Return the stock to the pan, add the reserved chillies and spring onions, the sugar, lime juice, coriander and salt to taste.

4 Simmer for 5 minutes, then add the carrot flowers and tofu, and cook for a further 2 minutes until the carrot is just tender. Serve hot.

HEALTH BENEFITS

Hot spices, including chillies, are good for the respiratory system. They help to relieve congestion and may, as a result, soothe the symptoms of colds, flu and hayfever. Chillies encourage the brain to release endorphins, which increase the sensation of pleasure, and so they have been described as aphrodisiacs.

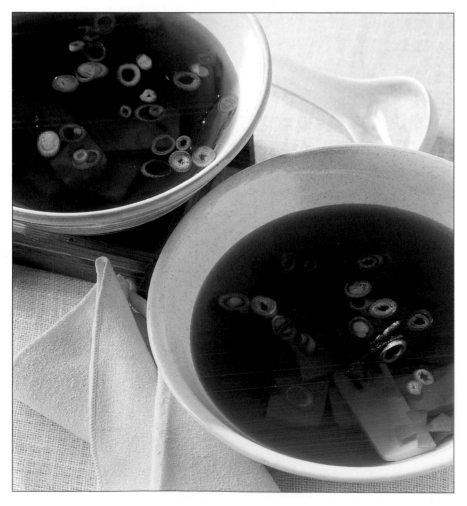

Roasted Root Vegetable Soup

ADAPT THE COMBINATION and quantities of seasonal vegetables used in this soup depending on what's available and to vary the balance of nutrients.

INGREDIENTS

50ml/2fl oz/¼ cup olive oil
1 small butternut squash, peeled, seeded and cubed
2 carrots, cut into thick rounds
1 large parsnip, cubed
1 small swede, cubed
2 leeks, thickly sliced
1 onion, quartered
3 bay leaves
4 thyme sprigs, plus extra to garnish
3 rosemary sprigs
1.2 litres/2 pints/5 cups vegetable stock
salt and freshly ground black pepper
soured cream, to serve
Serves 6

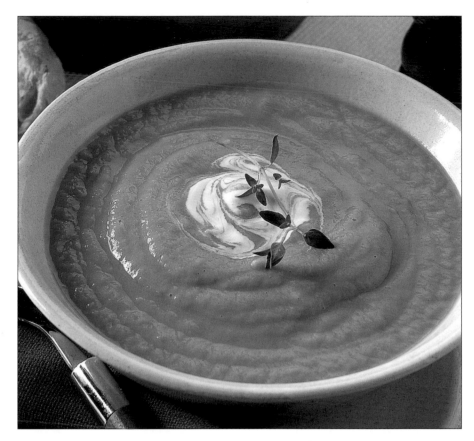

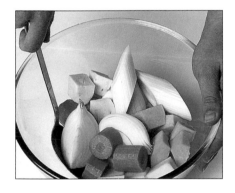
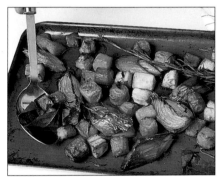
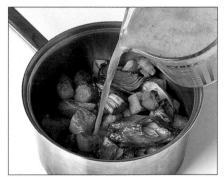

1 Preheat the oven to 200°C/400°F/ Gas 6. Put the olive oil into a large bowl. Add the prepared vegetables and toss until coated in the oil.

2 Spread out the vegetables in a single layer on one large or two small baking sheets. Tuck the bay leaves and thyme and rosemary sprigs amongst the vegetables.

COOK'S TIP

Dried herbs can be used in place of fresh; sprinkle 2.5ml/½ tsp of each type over the vegetables in step 2.

3 Roast the vegetables for about 50 minutes until tender, turning them occasionally to make sure they brown evenly. Remove from the oven, discard the herbs and transfer the vegetables to a large saucepan.

HEALTH BENEFITS

This nutritious soup is packed with health-giving vegetables. Butternut squash is particularly high in betacarotene and potassium, which is essential for the functioning of the cells, nerves and muscles. Carrots also contain a high level of beta-carotene and are effective detoxifiers.

4 Pour the stock into the pan and bring to the boil. Reduce the heat, season to taste, then simmer for 10 minutes. Transfer the soup to a food processor or blender (or use a hand blender) and process for a few minutes until thick and smooth.

5 Return the soup to the pan to heat through. Season and serve with a swirl of soured cream. Garnish each serving with a sprig of thyme.

Jerusalem Artichoke Soup with Gruyère Toasts

SMALL, KNOBBLY JERUSALEM artichokes have a delicious, mild, nutty flavour and make a wonderful, wholesome creamy soup. Each spoonful will give you the energy your body needs during cold winter days.

INGREDIENTS

30ml/2 tbsp olive oil
1 large onion, chopped
1 garlic clove, chopped
1 celery stick, chopped
675g/1 1/2lb jerusalem artichokes, peeled or scrubbed, and chopped
1.2 litres/2 pints/5 cups vegetable stock
300ml/1/2 pint/1 1/4 cups semi-skimmed milk
salt and freshly ground black pepper

To serve
8 slices French bread
115g/4oz/1 cup Gruyère cheese, grated
Serves 4–6

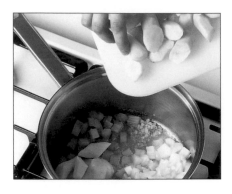

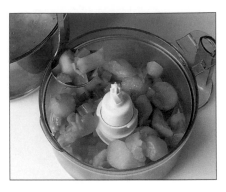

1 Heat the oil in a large saucepan. Add the onion, garlic and celery, and cook over a medium heat for about 5 minutes or until softened, stirring occasionally. Add the prepared jerusalem artichokes and cook for a further 5 minutes.

2 Add the stock and seasoning, then bring the soup to the boil. Reduce the heat and simmer for 20–25 minutes, stirring occasionally, until the artichokes are tender.

3 Transfer the soup to a food processor or blender (or use a hand blender) and process for a few minutes until smooth. Return the soup to the pan, stir in the milk and heat through gently for 2 minutes.

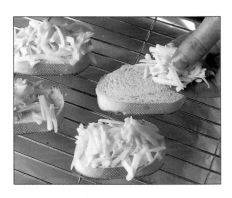

4 To make the Gruyère toasts, heat the grill to high. Lightly grill the bread on one side, then sprinkle the untoasted side with the Gruyère. Grill until the cheese melts and is golden. Ladle the soup into bowls and top with the Gruyère toasts.

COOK'S TIP

To preserve soluble nutrients, scrub the jerusalem artichokes rather than peel them.

HEALTH BENEFITS

High in fibre and low in fat, jerusalem artichokes also contain valuable amounts of vitamin C.

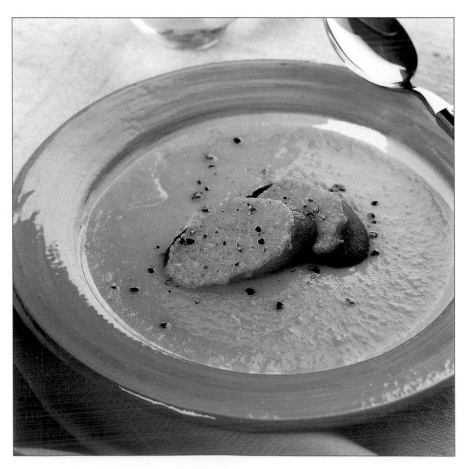

Thai Fish Broth

LEMON GRASS, CHILLIES AND GALANGAL add flavour this fragrant soup, and help to boost the immune system.

INGREDIENTS

1 litre/1¾ pints/4 cups fish or light
   vegetable stock
4 lemon grass stalks
3 limes
2 small fresh hot red chillies, seeded
   and thinly sliced
2cm/¾in piece fresh galangal, peeled
   and thinly sliced
6 coriander stalks, with leaves
2 kaffir lime leaves, coarsely
   chopped (optional)
350g/12oz monkfish fillet, skinned and
   cut into 2.5cm/1in pieces
15ml/1 tbsp rice vinegar
45ml/3 tbsp nam pla (Thai fish sauce)
30ml/2 tbsp chopped coriander leaves,
   to garnish

Serves 2–3

1 Pour the stock into a saucepan and bring it to the boil. Meanwhile, slice the bulb end of each lemon grass stalk diagonally into pieces about 3mm/⅛in thick. Peel off four wide strips of lime rind with a potato peeler, taking care to avoid the white pith underneath the skin which would make the soup bitter. Squeeze the limes and reserve the juice.

2 Add the sliced lemon grass, lime rind, chillies, galangal and coriander stalks to the stock, with the kaffir lime leaves, if using. Simmer for 1–2 minutes.

HEALTH BENEFITS

Chillies are an excellent source of vitamins C and E, folate and potassium. They can also help to stimulate the body and improve the circulation.

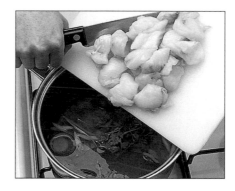

3 Add the pieces of monkfish, rice vinegar and nam pla, with about half the reserved lime juice. Simmer over a low heat for about 3 minutes, until the fish is just cooked.

4 Lift out and discard the coriander stalks, taste the broth and add more lime juice if necessary; the soup should taste quite sour, but not bitter. Ladle into individual bowls, sprinkle with the chopped coriander leaves and serve very hot.

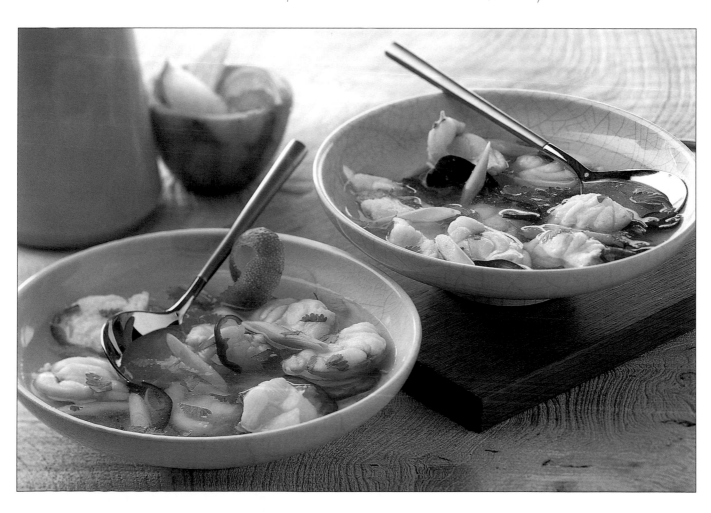

Aubergine, Smoked Mozzarella and Basil Rolls

SLICES OF GRILLED AUBERGINE stuffed with smoked mozzarella, tomato and fresh basil make an attractive hors-d'oeuvre, or a light lunch and provide the body with protein and essential vitamins and minerals.

INGREDIENTS

1 large aubergine
45ml/3 tbsp olive oil, plus extra for
   drizzling (optional)
165g/5¹/₂oz smoked mozzarella cheese,
   cut into 8 slices
2 plum tomatoes, each cut into 4 slices
8 large basil leaves
balsamic vinegar, for drizzling (optional)
salt and freshly ground black pepper
Serves 4

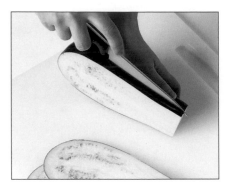

1 Cut the aubergine lengthways into 10 thin slices and discard the two outermost slices. Sprinkle the slices with salt and leave for 20 minutes. Rinse, then pat dry with kitchen paper.

2 Preheat the grill and line the rack with foil. Place the dried aubergine slices on the grill rack and brush liberally with oil. Grill for 8–10 minutes until tender and golden, turning once.

3 Remove the aubergine slices from the grill, then place a slice of mozzarella. a slice of tomato and a basil leaf in the centre of each and season to taste. Fold the aubergine over the filling and cook seam-side down under the grill until heated through and the mozzarella begins to melt. Serve drizzled with olive oil and a little balsamic vinegar, if using.

HEALTH BENEFITS

Aubergines are low in calories but frying will dramatically increase their calorific value. Salting the aubergine first not only draws out any bitter juices, it also makes the flesh denser, so that less fat is absorbed during cooking. Aubergines contain bioflavonoids, which help to prevent strokes and haemorrhages.

Creamy Lemon Puy Lentils

TINY, GREEN PUY LENTILS are an excellent source of low-fat protein and provide a steady release of energy that helps keep blood-sugar levels stable.

INGREDIENTS

250g/9oz/generous 1 cup Puy lentils
1 bay leaf
30ml/2 tbsp olive oil
4 spring onions, sliced
2 large garlic cloves, chopped
15ml/1 tbsp Dijon mustard
finely grated rind and juice of 1 large lemon
4 plum tomatoes, seeded and diced
4 eggs
60ml/4 tbsp crème fraîche
salt and freshly ground black pepper
30ml/2 tbsp chopped fresh flat leaf
   parsley, to garnish
Serves 4

1 Put the lentils and bay leaf in a saucepan, cover with cold water, and bring to the boil. Reduce the heat and simmer, partially covered, for 25 minutes or until the lentils are tender. Stir the lentils occasionally and add more water, if necessary. Drain.

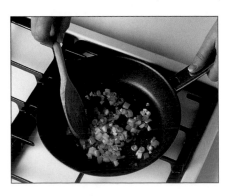

2 Heat the oil and fry the spring onions and garlic for 1 minute or until softened.

3 Add the Dijon mustard, lemon rind and juice, and mix well. Stir in the tomatoes and seasoning, then cook gently for 1–2 minutes until the tomatoes are heated through but still retain their shape. Add a little water if the mixture becomes too dry.

4 Meanwhile, poach the eggs in a saucepan of barely simmering salted water. Add the lentils and crème fraîche to the tomato mixture, remove the bay leaf, and heat through for 1 minute. Top each portion with a poached egg, and sprinkle with parsley.

HEALTH BENEFITS

Studies have shown that lentils may help prevent heart disease and cancer, and lower cholesterol levels.

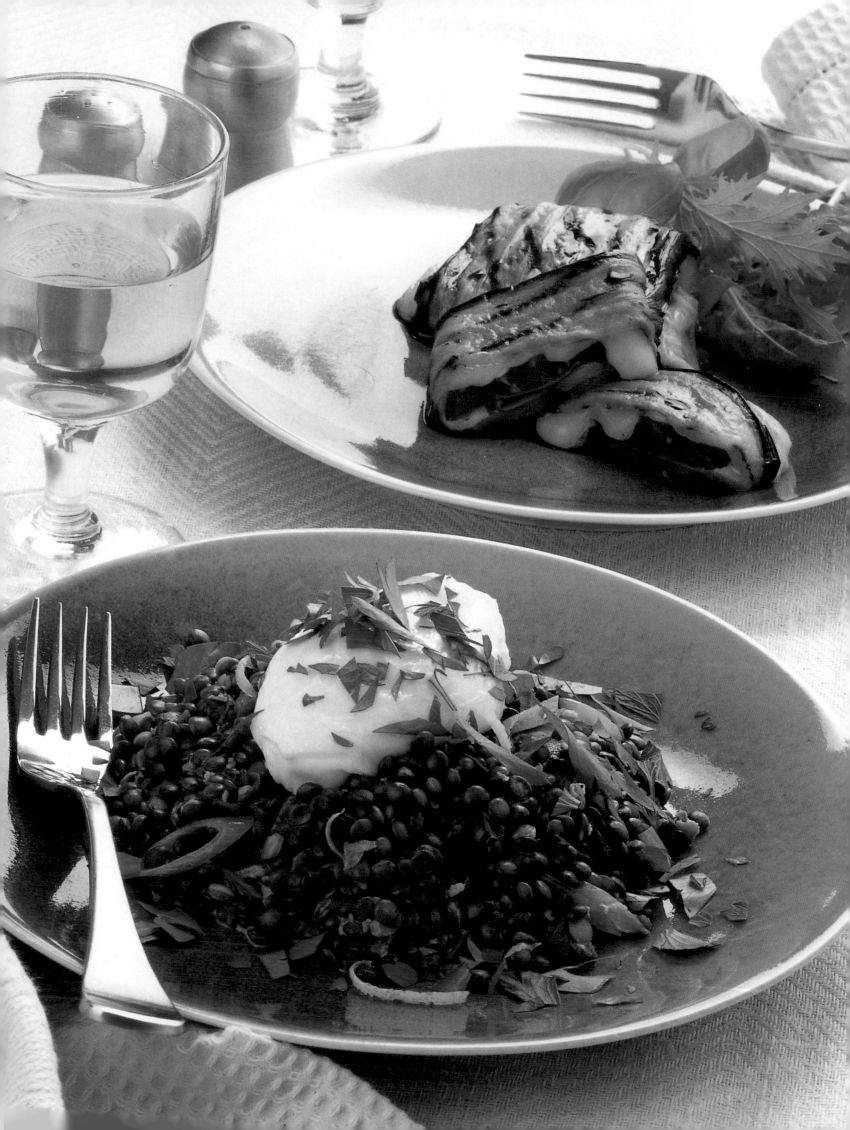

Thai Tempeh Cakes with Sweet Dipping Sauce

MADE FROM SOYA BEANS, TEMPEH is similar to tofu but has a nuttier taste. Here, it is combined with a fragrant blend of lemon grass, coriander and ginger and formed into small patties.

INGREDIENTS

1 lemon grass stalk, outer leaves removed
    and inside finely chopped
2 garlic cloves, chopped
2 spring onions, finely chopped
2 shallots, finely chopped
2 chillies, seeded and finely chopped
2.5cm/1in piece fresh root ginger,
    finely chopped
60ml/4 tbsp chopped fresh coriander, plus
    extra to garnish
250g/9oz/2¼ cups tempeh, defrosted if
    frozen, sliced
15ml/1 tbsp lime juice
5ml/1 tsp caster sugar
45ml/3 tbsp plain flour
1 large egg, lightly beaten
vegetable oil, for frying
salt and freshly ground black pepper

For the dipping sauce
45ml/3 tbsp mirin
45ml/3 tbsp white wine vinegar
2 spring onions, finely sliced
15ml/1 tbsp sugar
2 chillies, finely chopped
30ml/2 tbsp chopped fresh coriander
large pinch of salt
Makes 8

HEALTH BENEFITS

Although tempeh does not contain quite the same levels of calcium, iron and B vitamins as tofu, in many ways it is healthier. It is made from fermented whole soya beans and the mould used in the fermentation process is said to boost the immune system and free the body of harmful toxins.

1 To make the dipping sauce, mix together the mirin, vinegar, spring onions, sugar, chillies, coriander and salt in a small bowl and set aside.

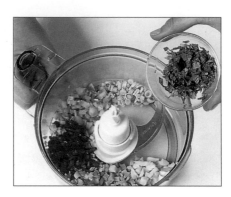

2 Place the lemon grass, garlic, spring onions, shallots, chillies, ginger and coriander in a food processor or blender, then process to a coarse paste. Add the tempeh, lime juice and sugar, then blend until combined. Add the seasoning, flour and egg. Process again until the mixture forms a coarse, sticky paste.

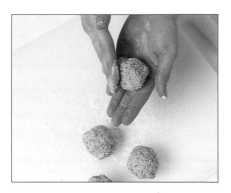

3 Take one-eighth of the tempeh mixture at a time and form into rounds with your hands – the mixture will be quite sticky.

4 Heat enough oil to cover the base of a large frying pan. Fry the tempeh cakes for 5–6 minutes, turning once, until golden. Drain on kitchen paper and serve warm with the dipping sauce, garnished with the reserved coriander.

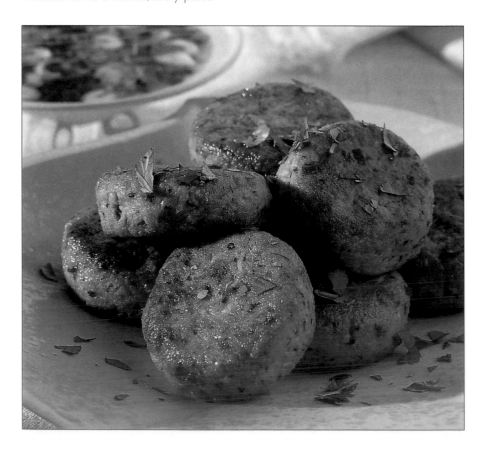

Cannellini Bean and Rosemary Bruschetta

MORE BRUNCH THAN BREAKFAST, this high-fibre dish is a sophisticated version of beans on toast.

INGREDIENTS

150g/5oz/2/3 cup dried cannellini beans
5 fresh tomatoes
45ml/3 tbsp olive oil, plus extra for drizzling
2 sun-dried tomatoes in oil, drained and
    finely chopped
1 garlic clove, crushed
30ml/2 tbsp chopped fresh rosemary
salt and freshly ground black pepper
a handful of fresh basil leaves, to garnish

To serve
12 slices Italian-style bread, such as ciabatta
1 large garlic clove, halved

Serves 4

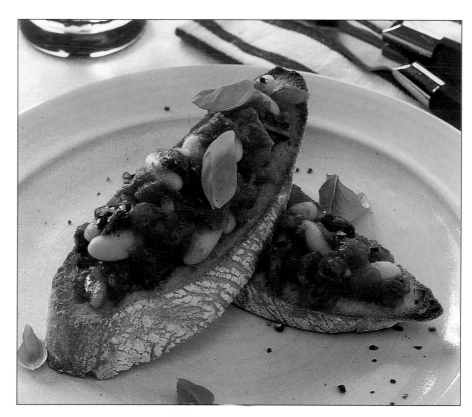

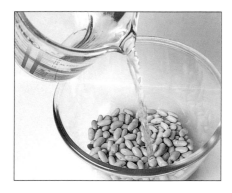

1 Place the beans in a large bowl and cover with water. Leave to soak overnight. Drain and rinse the beans, then place in a saucepan and cover with fresh water. Bring to the boil and boil rapidly for 10 minutes. Reduce the heat and simmer for 50–60 minutes or until tender. Drain and set aside.

2 Meanwhile, place the tomatoes in a bowl, cover with boiling water, leave for 30 seconds, then peel, seed and chop the flesh. Heat the oil in a frying pan, add the fresh and sun-dried tomatoes, garlic and rosemary. Cook for 2 minutes until the tomatoes begin to break down and soften.

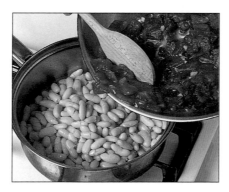

3 Add the tomato mixture to the cannellini beans, season to taste and mix well.

HEALTH BENEFITS

• Cannellini beans are high in protein and low in fat. They are also a valuable source of B vitamins and minerals.
• Rosemary is reputed to have many healing qualities. It is said to alleviate headaches, to improve the circulation and to ease rheumatism. Use fresh rosemary if possible, as dried will have lost most of its beneficial oils.

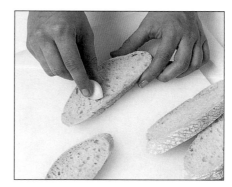

4 Rub the cut sides of the bread slices with the garlic clove, then toast lightly. Spoon the cannellini bean mixture on top of the toast. Sprinkle with basil leaves and drizzle with a little extra olive oil before serving.

COOK'S TIP

Canned beans can be used instead of dried; use 275g/10oz/2 cups drained, canned beans and add to the tomato mixture in step 3. If the beans are canned in brine, then rinse and drain them well before use.

Tortilla Wrap with Tabbouleh and Guacamole

THIS CLASSIC MIDDLE EASTERN salad is made with plenty of spring onions, lemon juice, fresh herbs and lots of freshly ground black pepper, which can help to promote good health, provide energy and help the body to fight illness.

INGREDIENTS

175g/6oz/1 cup bulgur wheat
30ml/2 tbsp chopped fresh mint
30ml/2 tbsp chopped fresh flat
  leaf parsley
1 bunch spring onions (about 6), sliced
1/2 cucumber, diced
50ml/2fl oz/1/4 cup extra virgin olive oil
juice of 1 large lemon
salt and freshly ground black pepper
4 wheat tortillas, to serve
flat leaf parsley, to garnish (optional)

For the guacamole
1 ripe avocado, stoned, peeled and diced
juice of 1/2 lemon
1/2 red chilli, seeded and sliced
1 garlic clove, crushed
1/2 red pepper, seeded and finely diced
Serves 4–6

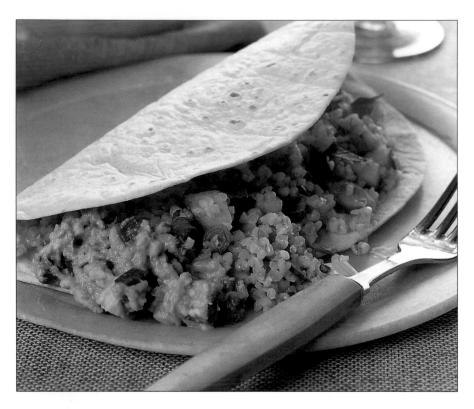

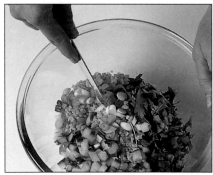

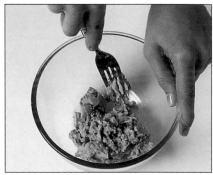

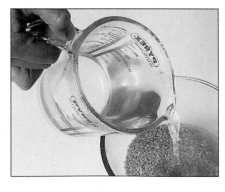

1 To make the tabbouleh, place the bulgur wheat in a large heatproof bowl and pour over enough boiling water to cover. Leave for 30 minutes until the grains are tender but still retain a little resistance to the bite. Drain thoroughly in a sieve, then tip back into the bowl.

2 Add the mint, parsley, spring onions and cucumber to the bulgur wheat and mix thoroughly. Blend together the olive oil and lemon juice and pour over the tabbouleh, season to taste and toss well to mix. Chill for 30 minutes to allow the flavours to mingle.

COOK'S TIP

The soaking time for bulgur wheat can vary. For the best results, follow the instructions on the packet and taste the grain every now and again to check whether it is tender enough.

3 To make the guacamole, place the avocado in a bowl and add the lemon juice, chilli and garlic. Season to taste and mash with a fork to form a smooth purée. Stir in the red pepper.

4 Warm the tortillas in a dry frying pan and serve either flat, folded or rolled up with the tabbouleh and guacamole. Garnish with parsley, if using.

HEALTH BENEFITS

• *Bulgur wheat is a useful source of dietary fibre and B complex vitamins.*
• *Parsley and mint are good digestives.*

Ceviche

THIS SOUTH AMERICAN DISH combines nutritious fish with vitamin C-rich chillies and limes.

INGREDIENTS

675g/1½ lb halibut, turbot, sea bass or
*   salmon fillets, skinned*
juice of 3 limes
1–2 fresh red chillies, seeded and very
*   finely chopped*
15ml/1 tbsp olive oil
salt

For the garnish

4 large firm tomatoes, peeled, seeded
*   and diced*
1 ripe avocado, peeled
*   and diced*
15ml/1 tbsp lemon juice
30ml/2 tbsp olive oil
30ml/2 tbsp fresh coriander leaves
Serves 6

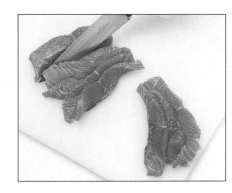

1 Cut the fish into strips measuring about 5 × 1cm/2 × ½in. Lay these in a shallow, non-metallic dish and pour over the lime juice, turning the fish strips to coat them all over in the juice. Cover with clear film and set aside for at least 1 hour.

2 To make the garnish, gently mix together the diced tomatoes, avocado, lemon juice and olive oil in a medium bowl. Set aside.

3 Season the fish to taste with salt and scatter over the chopped chillies. Drizzle with the olive oil. Toss the fish in the mixture, then cover again with clear film. Set aside in the fridge to marinate for a further 15–30 minutes.

4 To serve, divide the garnish among six individual plates. Spoon on the ceviche, sprinkle with coriander leaves and serve.

HEALTH BENEFITS

Oily fish, such as salmon, provide an excellent supply of omega-3 fatty acids, which have been found to help reduce the risk of heart disease, blood clots and strokes. Omega-3 fatty acids are also thought to help regulate blood pressure.

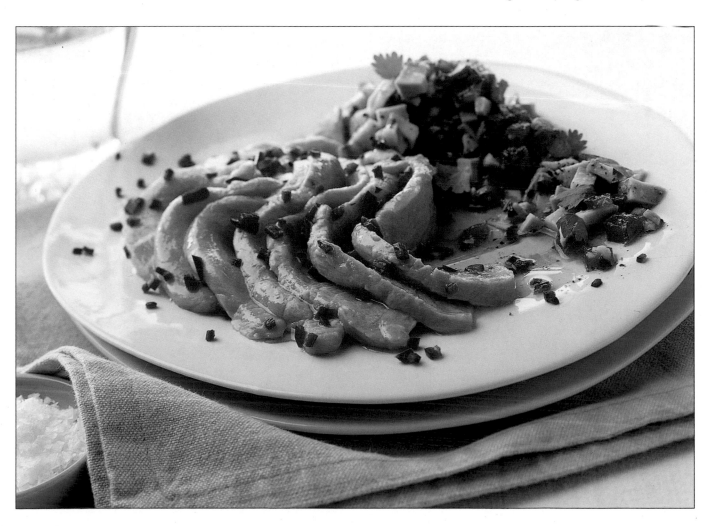

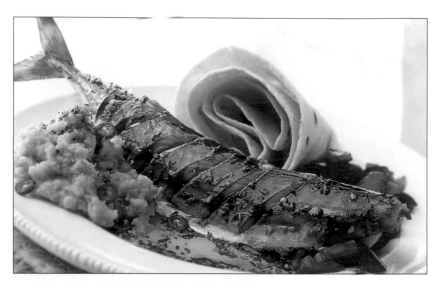

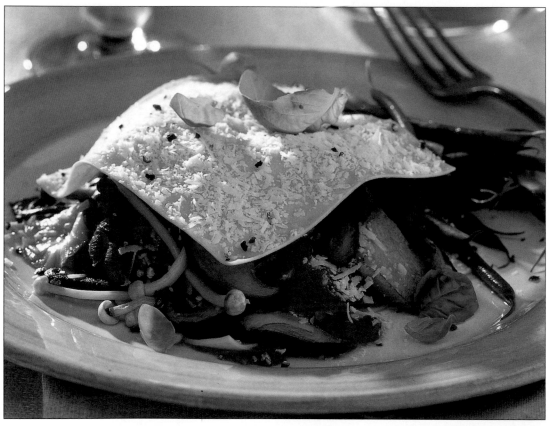

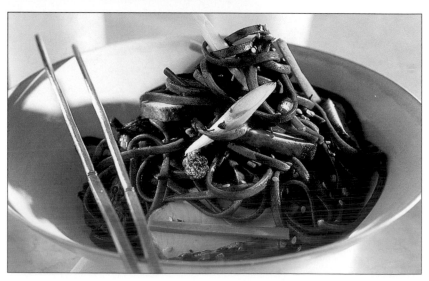

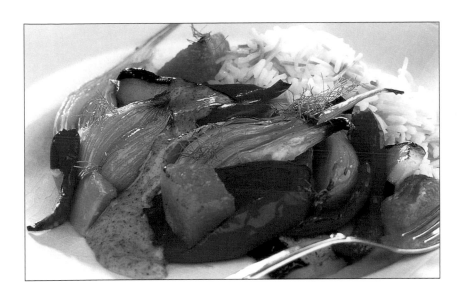

MAIN DISHES

The recipes in this chapter are mainly carbohydrate-based, incorporating pulses, such as beans and lentils, and pasta and rice. These foods are filling, packed with fibre, vitamins and minerals, and supply valuable low-fat protein. Included are some of the most innovative main-course dishes on anybody's menu, from Thai Vegetable Curry with Lemon Grass Rice to Roasted Vegetables with Salsa Verde. Dishes such as Grilled Mackerel with Spicy Dhal, and Pappardelle, Sardine and Fennel Bake also offer a good source of essential fatty acids.

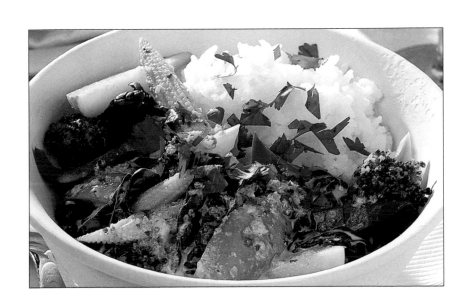

Thai Vegetable Curry with Lemon Grass Rice

FRAGRANT JASMINE RICE, subtly flavoured with lemon grass and cardamom, is the perfect accompaniment to this richly spiced vegetable curry. The combination of spices and fresh vegetables offers a wealth of goodness.

INGREDIENTS

10ml/2 tsp vegetable oil

400ml/14fl oz/1²/3 cups coconut milk

300ml/¹/2 pint/1¹/4 cups vegetable stock

225g/8oz new potatoes, halved or
  quartered, if large

130g/4¹/2oz baby corn cobs

5ml/1 tsp golden caster sugar

185g/6¹/2oz broccoli florets

1 red pepper, seeded and sliced lengthways

115g/4oz spinach, tough stalks removed
  and shredded

30ml/2 tbsp chopped fresh coriander

salt and freshly ground black pepper

For the spice paste

1 red chilli, seeded and chopped

3 green chillies, seeded and chopped

1 lemon grass stalk, outer leaves removed
  and lower 5cm/2in finely chopped

2 shallots, chopped

finely grated rind of 1 lime

2 garlic cloves, chopped

5ml/1 tsp ground coriander

2.5ml/¹/2 tsp ground cumin

1cm/¹/2in fresh galangal, finely chopped or
  2.5ml/¹/2 tsp dried (optional)

30ml/2 tbsp chopped fresh coriander

15ml/1 tbsp chopped fresh coriander roots
  and stems (optional)

For the rice

225g/8oz/generous 1 cup jasmine
  rice, rinsed

1 lemon grass stalk, outer leaves removed
  and cut into 3 pieces

6 cardamom pods, bruised

Serves 4

1 Make the spice paste. Place all the ingredients in a food processor or blender and blend to a coarse paste.

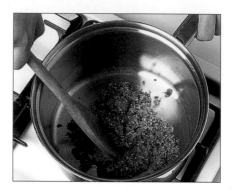

2 Heat the oil in a large heavy-based saucepan and fry the spice paste for 1–2 minutes, stirring constantly. Add the coconut milk and stock, and bring to the boil.

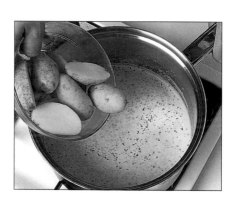

3 Reduce the heat, add the potatoes and simmer for 15 minutes. Add the baby corn and seasoning, then cook for 2 minutes. Stir in the sugar, broccoli and red pepper, and cook for 2 minutes more until the vegetables are tender. Stir in the shredded spinach and half the fresh coriander. Cook for 2 minutes.

HEALTH BENEFITS

Broccoli provides valuable amounts of calcium, vitamin C, folic acid, zinc and iron. The vitamin and mineral content of this dish is given a further boost by the addition of all the other vegetables.

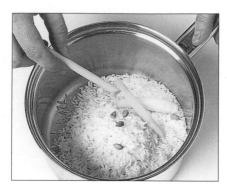

4 Meanwhile, prepare the lemon grass rice. Tip the rinsed rice into a large saucepan and add the lemon grass and cardamom pods. Pour over 475ml/16fl oz/2 cups water.

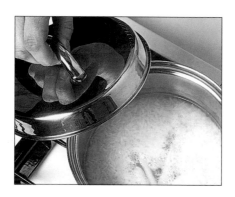

5 Bring to the boil, then reduce the heat, cover, and cook for 10–15 minutes until the water is absorbed and the rice is tender and slightly sticky. Season with salt, leave to stand for 10 minutes, then fluff up the rice with a fork.

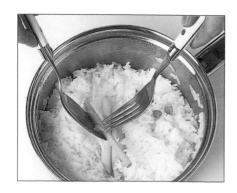

6 Remove the spices and serve the rice with the curry, sprinkled with the remaining fresh coriander.

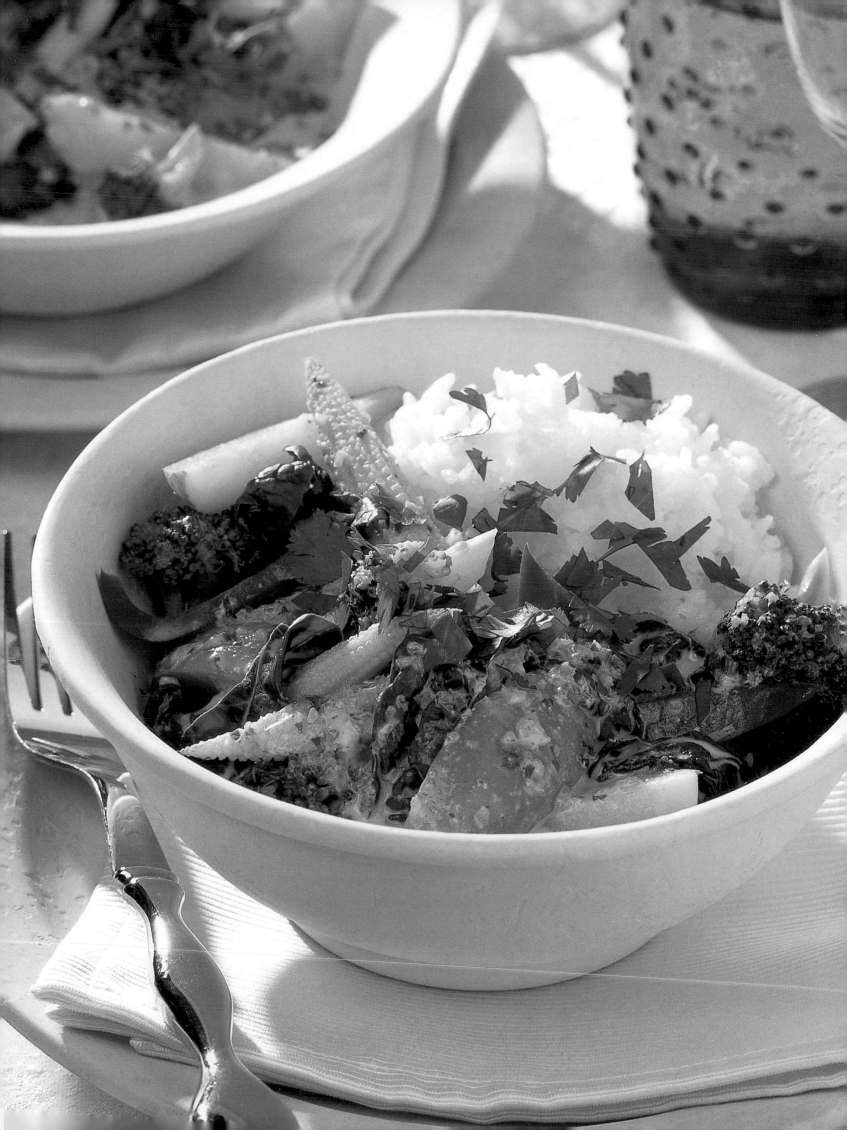

Potato Rösti and Tofu with Fresh Tomato and Ginger Sauce

ALTHOUGH THIS DISH FEATURES various components, it is not difficult to make and the finished result is well worth the effort. Tofu is rich in isoflavones and is believed to help with a number of health conditions. To name but a few, it is thought to help lower blood cholesterol levels, ease arthritis and reduce the risk of osteoporosis.

INGREDIENTS

425g/15oz/3³/4 cups tofu, cut into
   1cm/¹/2in cubes
4 large potatoes, about 900g/2lb total
   weight, peeled
sunflower oil, for frying
salt and freshly ground black pepper
30ml/2 tbsp sesame seeds, toasted

For the marinade
30ml/2 tbsp tamari or dark soy sauce
15ml/1 tbsp clear honey
2 garlic cloves, crushed
4 cm/1¹/2 in piece fresh root ginger, grated
5ml/1 tsp toasted sesame oil

For the sauce
15ml/1 tbsp olive oil
8 tomatoes, halved, seeded and chopped
Serves 4

1 Mix together all the marinade ingredients in a shallow dish and add the tofu. Spoon the marinade over the tofu and leave to marinate in the fridge for at least 1 hour. Turn the tofu occasionally in the marinade to allow the flavours to infuse.

HEALTH BENEFITS

Made from processed soya beans, tofu is a highly nutritious protein food and is the richest non-dairy source of calcium. Tofu also contains valuable B complex vitamins and iron.

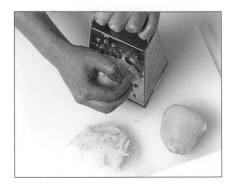

2 To make the rösti, par-boil the potatoes for 10–15 minutes until almost tender. Leave to cool, then grate coarsely. Season well. Preheat the oven to 200°C/400°F/Gas 6.

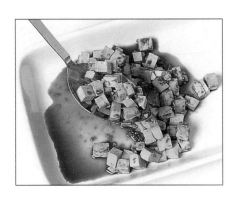

3 Using a slotted spoon, remove the tofu from the marinade and reserve the marinade. Spread out the tofu on a baking tray and bake for 20 minutes, turning occasionally, until golden and crisp on all sides.

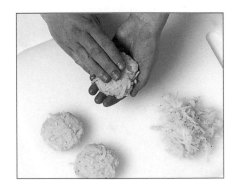

4 Take a quarter of the potato mixture in your hands at a time and form into rough cakes.

5 Heat a frying pan with just enough oil to cover the base. Place the cakes in the frying pan and flatten the mixture, using your hands or a spatula to form rounds about 1cm/¹/2in thick.

6 Cook for about 6 minutes until golden and crisp underneath. Carefully turn over the rösti and cook for a further 6 minutes until golden.

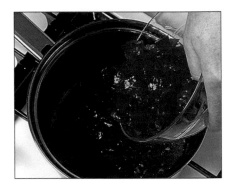

7 Meanwhile, make the sauce. Heat the oil in a saucepan, add the reserved marinade and the tomatoes and cook for 2 minutes, stirring. Reduce the heat and simmer, covered, for 10 minutes, stirring occasionally, until the tomatoes break down. Press through a sieve to make a thick, smooth sauce.

8 To serve, place a rösti on each of four warm serving plates. Scatter the tofu on top, spoon over the tomato sauce and sprinkle with sesame seeds.

COOK'S TIP

Tamari is a thick, mellow-flavoured Japanese soy sauce, which unlike conventional Chinese soy sauce is wheat-free, and so is suitable for people who are on wheat- or gluten-free diets. It is sold in Japanese food shops and some larger health food stores.

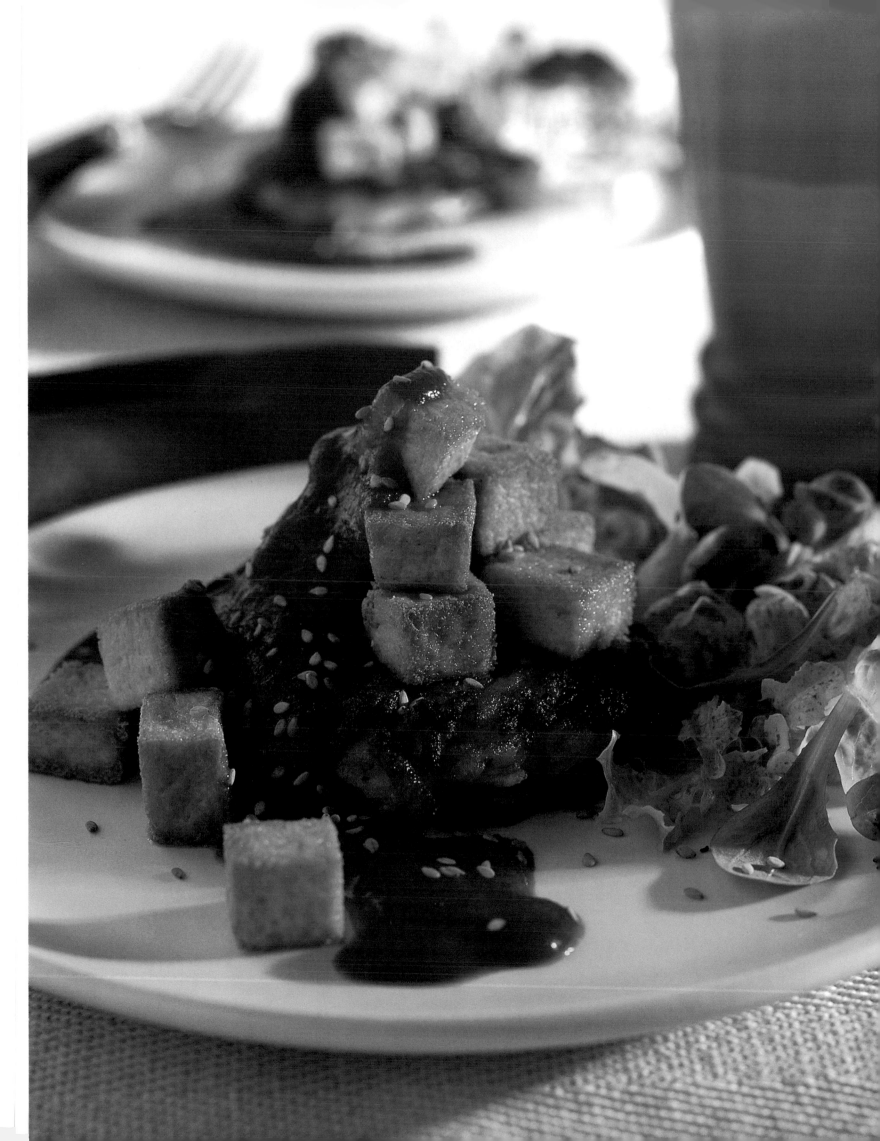

Roasted Vegetables with Salsa Verde

THERE ARE ENDLESS VARIATIONS of the Italian salsa verde, which means "green sauce". Usually a blend of fresh chopped herbs, garlic, olive oil, anchovies and capers, this is a simplified version that offers all the goodness of these fresh ingredients and makes the perfect partner for vegetables.

INGREDIENTS

3 courgettes, sliced lengthways
1 large fennel bulb, cut into wedges
450g/1lb butternut squash, cut into
    2cm/3/4in chunks
12 shallots
2 red peppers, seeded and cut lengthways
    into thick slices
4 plum tomatoes, halved and seeded
45ml/3 tbsp olive oil
2 garlic cloves, crushed
5ml/1 tsp balsamic vinegar
salt and freshly ground black pepper

For the salsa verde
45ml/3 tbsp chopped fresh mint
90ml/6 tbsp chopped fresh flat leaf
    parsley
15ml/1 tbsp Dijon mustard
juice of 1/2 lemon
30ml/2 tbsp olive oil

For the rice
15ml/1 tbsp vegetable or olive oil
75g/3oz/3/4 cup vermicelli, broken into
    short lengths
225g/8oz/generous 1 cup long grain rice
900ml/1 1/2 pints/3 3/4 cups vegetable stock
Serves 4

COOK'S TIP

The salsa verde will keep for up to
1 week if stored in an airtight container
in the fridge.

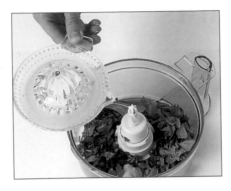

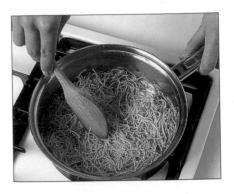

1 Preheat the oven to 220°C/425°F/ Gas 7. To make the salsa verde, place all the ingredients, with the exception of the olive oil, in a food processor or blender. Blend to a coarse paste, then add the oil, a little at a time, until the mixture forms a smooth purée. Season to taste.

2 To roast the vegetables, toss the courgettes, fennel, squash, shallots, peppers and tomatoes in the olive oil, garlic and balsamic vinegar. Leave for 10 minutes to allow the flavours to mingle.

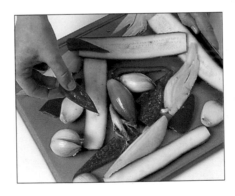

3 Place all the vegetables – apart from the squash and tomatoes – on a baking sheet, brush with half the oil and vinegar mixture and season.

4 Roast for 25 minutes, then remove the tray from the oven. Turn the vegetables over and brush with the rest of the oil and vinegar mixture. Add the squash and tomatoes and cook for a further 20–25 minutes until all the vegetables are tender and lightly blackened around the edges.

5 Meanwhile, prepare the rice. Heat the oil in a heavy-based saucepan. Add the vermicelli and fry for about 3 minutes or until golden and crisp. Season to taste.

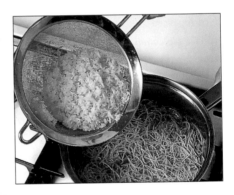

6 Rinse the rice under cold running water, then drain well and add it to the vermicelli. Cook for 1 minute, stirring to coat it in the oil.

7 Add the vegetable stock, then cover the pan and cook for about 12 minutes until the water is absorbed. Stir the rice, then cover and leave to stand for 10 minutes. Serve the warm rice with the roasted vegetables and salsa verde.

HEALTH BENEFITS

• Brightly coloured vegetables, such as peppers, tomatoes and courgettes, are packed with the antioxidant vitamins C and E, and betacarotene, which are thought to reduce the risk of cancer.
• Mint aids the digestion and can help anyone who is suffering from irritable bowel syndrome.

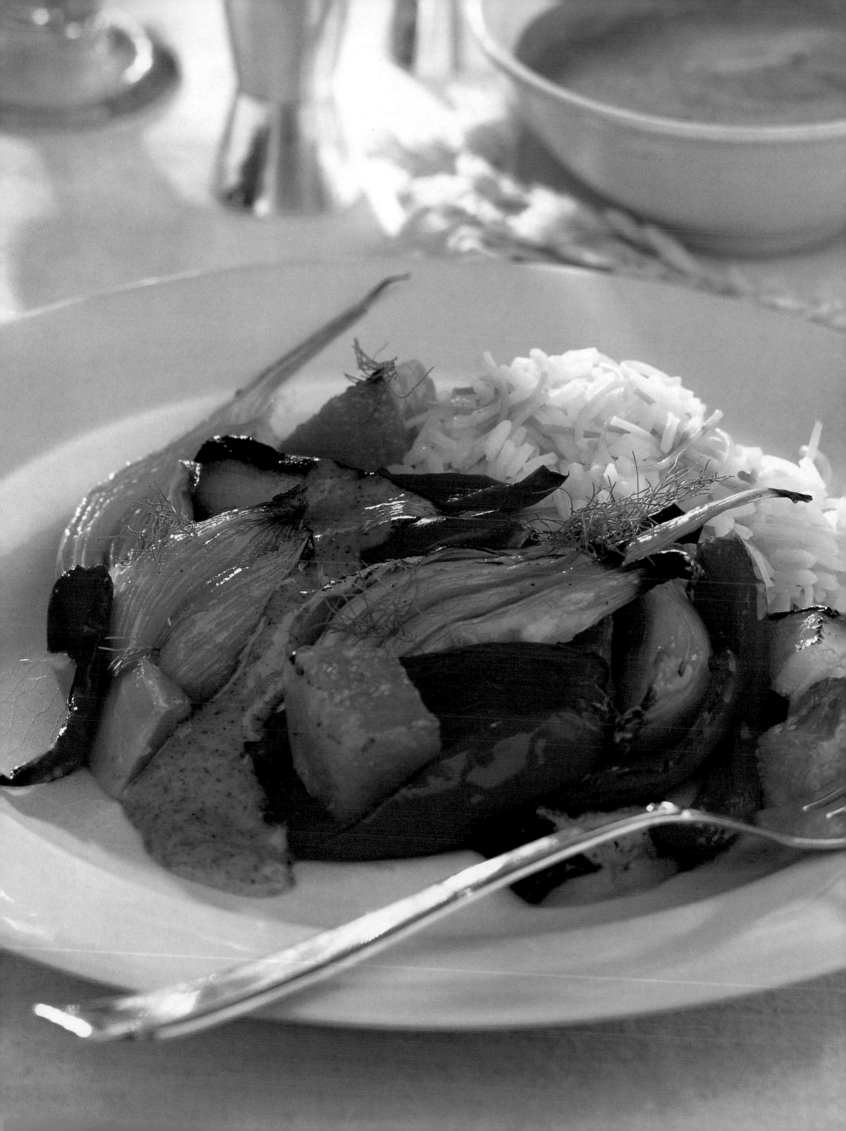

Grilled Mackerel with Spicy Dhal

OILY FISH, such as mackerel, are an important part of the diet and should be eaten two or three times a week.

INGREDIENTS

250g/9oz/1 cup red lentils, or yellow split peas (soaked overnight)
1 litre/1¾ pints/4 cups water
30ml/2 tbsp sunflower oil
2.5ml/½ tsp each mustard seeds, cumin seeds, fennel seeds, and fenugreek or cardamom seeds
5ml/1 tsp ground turmeric
3–4 dried red chillies, crumbled
30ml/2 tbsp tamarind paste
5ml/1 tsp soft brown sugar
30ml/2 tbsp chopped fresh coriander
4 mackerel or 8 large sardines
salt and ground black pepper
fresh red chilli slices and finely chopped coriander, to garnish
flat bread and tomatoes, to serve

Serves 4

1 Rinse the lentils or split peas, drain them thoroughly and put them in a saucepan. Pour in the water and bring to the boil over a medium heat. (Do not add salt or they will become tough.) Lower the heat, partially cover the pan and simmer the pulses for 30–40 minutes, stirring occasionally, until they are tender and mushy.

2 Heat the oil in a wok or shallow pan. Add the mustard seeds, then cover and cook for a few seconds, until they pop and give off their aroma. Remove the lid, add the rest of the seeds, with the turmeric and chillies and fry for a few more seconds.

3 Stir in the pulses, with salt to taste. Mix well; stir in the tamarind paste and sugar. Bring to the boil, then simmer for 10 minutes, until thick. Stir in the chopped fresh coriander.

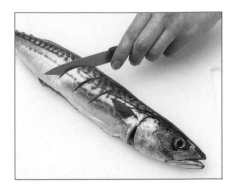

4 Meanwhile, clean the fish, then heat a ridged griddle or preheat the grill until very hot. Make six diagonal slashes on either side of each fish and remove the head if you wish. Season to taste with salt and pepper inside and out.

5 Grill the fish for 5–7 minutes on each side, until the skin is crisp. Serve with the dhal, flat bread and tomatoes, garnished with red chilli and chopped coriander.

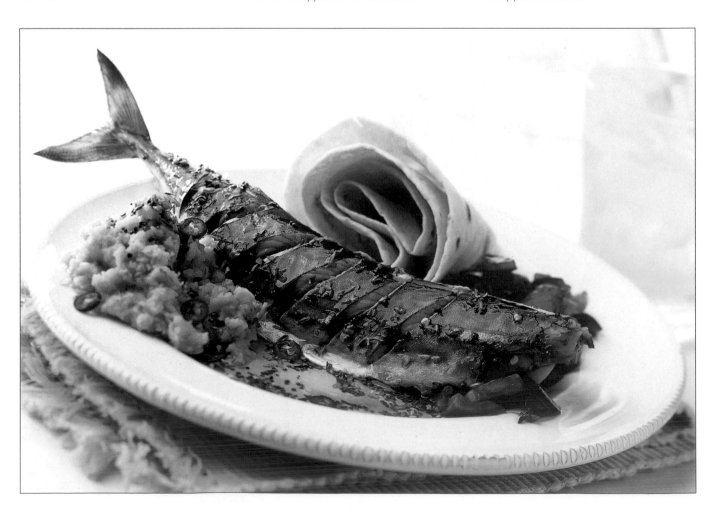

Oriental Fish en Papillote

THIS HEALTHY AROMATIC dish provides an excellent supply of essential fatty acids, vitamins and minerals, which can help to fight against cancer and other serious diseases as well as boosting the immune system.

INGREDIENTS

2 carrots

2 courgettes

6 spring onions

2.5cm/1in piece fresh root
   ginger, peeled

1 lime

2 garlic cloves, thinly sliced

30ml/2 tbsp teriyaki marinade or nam pla
   (Thai fish sauce)

5–10ml/1–2 tsp clear sesame oil

4 salmon fillets, about
   200g/7oz each

ground black pepper

rice, to serve

Serves 4

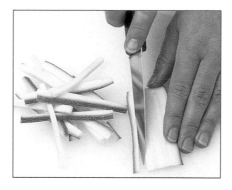

1 Cut the carrots, courgettes and spring onions into matchsticks and set them aside. Cut the ginger into matchsticks and put these in a small bowl. Using a zester, pare the lime thinly. Add the pared rind to the ginger, together with the garlic slices. Squeeze the lime juice.

2 Pour the teriyaki marinade or nam pla into a non-metallic bowl and stir in the lime juice and sesame oil until thoroughly combined.

3 Preheat the oven to 220°C/ 425°F/Gas 7. Cut out four rounds of non-stick baking paper, each with a diameter of 40cm/16in. Season the salmon to taste with pepper. Lay a fillet on one side of each paper round, about 3cm/1¼in off-centre. Scatter a quarter of the ginger mixture over each and pile a quarter of the vegetable matchsticks on top. Spoon a quarter of the teriyaki or nam pla mixture over the top.

4 Fold the bare side of the baking paper over the salmon and roll the edges of the paper over to seal each parcel very tightly.

5 Place the salmon parcels on a baking sheet and cook in the oven for 10–12 minutes, depending on the thickness of the fillets. Put the parcels on plates and serve with rice.

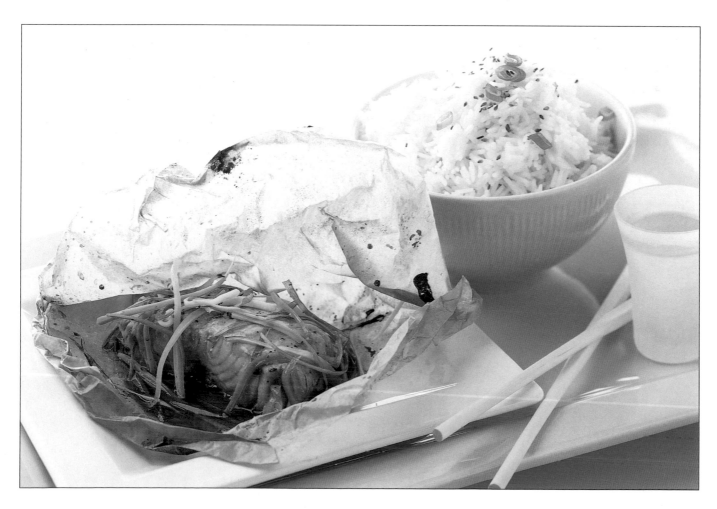

Baked Sea Bream with Tomatoes

FISH, SUCH AS SEA BREAM, is an excellent source of low-fat protein. If you prefer to use filleted fish, choose a chunky fillet, such as cod, and roast it skin side up.

INGREDIENTS

8 ripe tomatoes

10ml/2 tsp caster sugar

200ml/7fl oz/scant 1 cup olive oil

450g/1lb new potatoes

1 lemon, sliced

1 bay leaf

1 fresh thyme sprig

8 fresh basil leaves

1 sea bream, about 900g–1kg/
    2–2¼ lb, cleaned and scaled

150ml/¼ pint/⅔ cup dry white wine

30ml/2 tbsp fresh white breadcrumbs

2 garlic cloves, crushed

15ml/1 tbsp finely chopped fresh parsley

salt and ground black pepper

fresh flat leaf parsley or basil leaves,
    chopped, to garnish

Serves 4–6

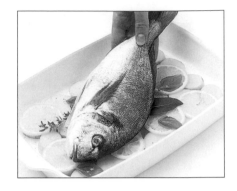

1 Preheat the oven to 240°C/475°F/ Gas 9. Cut the tomatoes in half lengthways and arrange them in a single layer in an ovenproof dish, cut side up. Sprinkle with sugar, salt and pepper and drizzle over a little of the olive oil. Roast for 30–40 minutes, until soft and lightly browned.

2 Meanwhile, cut the potatoes into 1cm/½in slices. Par-boil for about 5 minutes. Drain and set aside.

HEALTH BENEFITS

• Tomatoes are rich in vitamin C and contain the bioflavonoid lycopene, which is believed to prevent some forms of cancer by reducing the effects of harmful free radicals.

• Herbs have been highly prized by natural practitioners for centuries because, in spite of their low nutritional value, they possess many reputed healing qualities.

3 Brush an ovenproof dish with oil. Arrange the potatoes in a single layer with the lemon slices on top. Scatter over the bay leaf, thyme and basil. Season and drizzle with half the remaining olive oil. Lay the fish on top, season to taste and pour over the wine and the rest of the oil. Arrange the tomatoes around the fish.

4 Combine the breadcrumbs, garlic and parsley and sprinkle over the fish. Bake for 30 minutes, until the flesh comes away easily from the bone. Garnish with chopped parsley or basil.

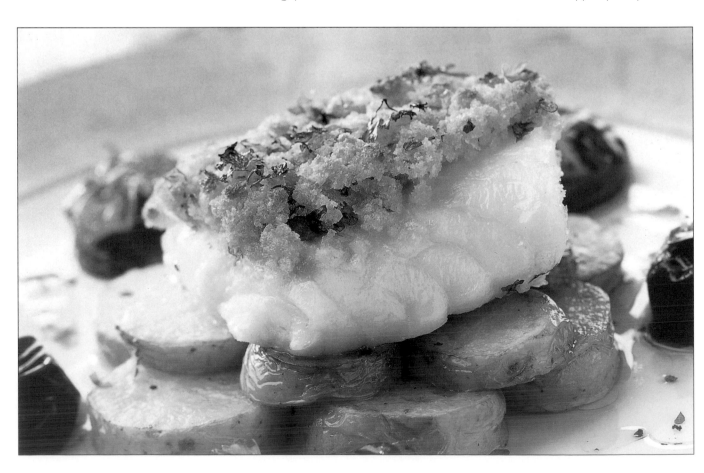

Pappardelle, Sardine and Fennel Bake

THE WIDE, FLAT NOODLES called pappardelle are perfect for this Sicilian recipe. If you can't find them, any wide pasta such as bucatini will do instead. Sardines are an excellent choice of fish as they are rich in essential fatty acids.

INGREDIENTS

2 fennel bulbs, trimmed
a large pinch of saffron threads
12 sardines, backbones and
    heads removed
60ml/4 tbsp olive oil
2 shallots, finely chopped
2 garlic cloves, finely chopped
2 fresh red chillies, seeded and
    finely chopped
4 drained canned anchovy fillets, or
    8–12 stoned black olives, chopped
30ml/2 tbsp capers
75g/3oz/¼ cup pine nuts
450g/1lb pappardelle
butter, for greasing
30ml/2 tbsp grated Pecorino cheese
salt and ground black pepper
Serves 6

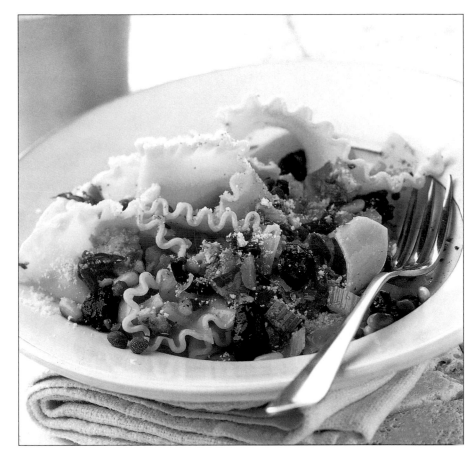

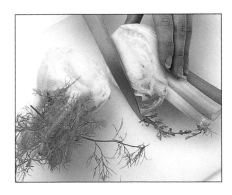

I Preheat the oven to 200°C/400°F/ Gas 6. Cut the fennel bulbs in half lengthways and cook them in a pan of lightly salted boiling water together with the saffron threads for about 10 minutes, until tender. Drain well, reserving the cooking liquid, and cut the fennel into small dice. Then finely chop the sardines, season to taste with salt and ground black pepper and set aside until required.

2 Heat the olive oil in a saucepan. Add the shallots and garlic and cook, stirring occasionally, until lightly coloured. Add the chillies and sardines and fry for 3 minutes. Stir in the fennel and cook over a low heat, stirring occasionally, for 3 minutes. If the mixture seems dry, add a little of the reserved fennel water.

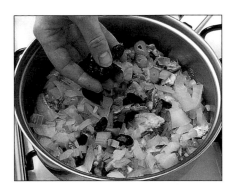

3 Add the anchovies or olives and cook for 1 minute. Stir in the capers and pine nuts, and season to taste with salt and pepper. Simmer for 3 minutes more, then turn off the heat.

4 Meanwhile, pour the reserved fennel liquid into a saucepan and top it up with enough water to cook the pasta. Stir in a little salt, bring to the boil and add the pappardelle. Cook dried pasta for about 12 minutes; fresh pasta until it rises to the surface of the water. When it is just tender, drain it.

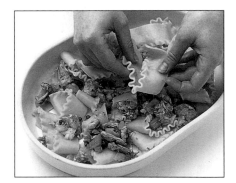

5 Grease a shallow ovenproof dish and put in a layer of pasta then make a layer of the sardine mixture. Continue making layers, finishing with the fish. Sprinkle over the Pecorino and bake for 15 minutes, until bubbling.

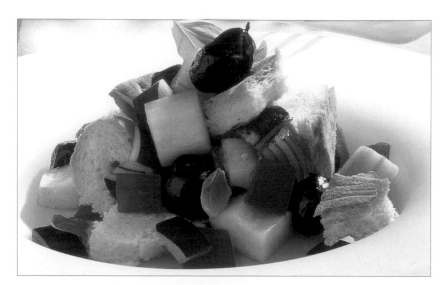

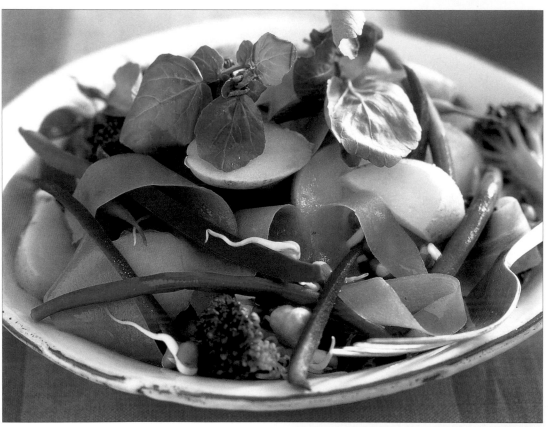

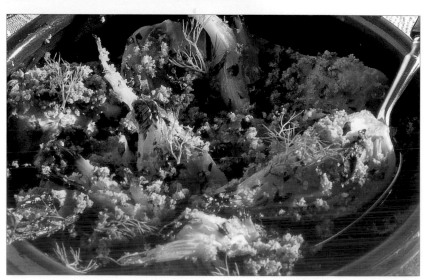

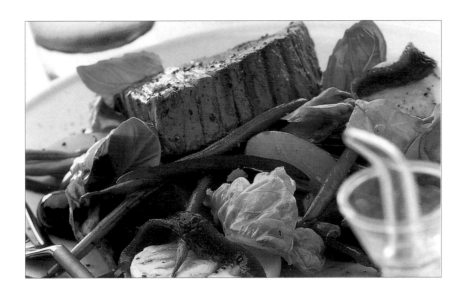

SALADS AND
SIDE DISHES

The recipes in this chapter are packed with fresh ingredients that

are highly valued for their cancer-thwarting phytochemicals,

antioxidants, vitamins, minerals and fibre. Try Avocado, Red Onion

and Spinach Salad with Polenta Croûtons, Courgettes in Rich

Tomato Sauce or Spring Vegetable Stir-fry to boost your intake

of these health-giving nutrients.

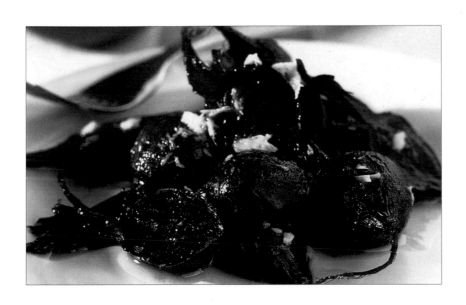

Warm Vegetable Salad with Peanut Sauce

BASED ON THE CLASSIC Indonesian salad, gado-gado, this dish combines nutritious raw red pepper and sprouted beans with lightly steamed broccoli, green beans and carrots and is topped with a spicy peanut sauce that is packed with health-promoting spices, including garlic, ginger and chillies.

INGREDIENTS

8 new potatoes
225g/8oz broccoli, cut into small florets
200g/7oz/1½ cups fine green beans
2 carrots, cut into thin ribbons with a
   vegetable peeler
1 red pepper, seeded and cut into strips
50g/2oz/½ cup sprouted beans
sprigs of watercress, to garnish

For the peanut sauce
15ml/1 tbsp sunflower oil
1 bird's eye chilli, seeded and sliced
1 garlic clove, crushed
5ml/1 tsp ground coriander
5ml/1 tsp ground cumin
60ml/4 tbsp crunchy peanut butter
75ml/5 tbsp water
15ml/1 tbsp dark soy sauce
1cm/½in piece fresh root ginger,
   finely grated
5ml/1 tsp soft dark brown sugar
15ml/1 tbsp lime juice
60ml/4 tbsp coconut milk
Serves 2–4

HEALTH BENEFITS

Sprouted beans, which are available from health food shops and some supermarkets, are easily digestible and packed with concentrated goodness. When fresh, their vitamin and enzyme content is at its peak and they are believed to stimulate the body's ability to cleanse itself. They provide valuable amounts of vitamin E, which is said to improve fertility.

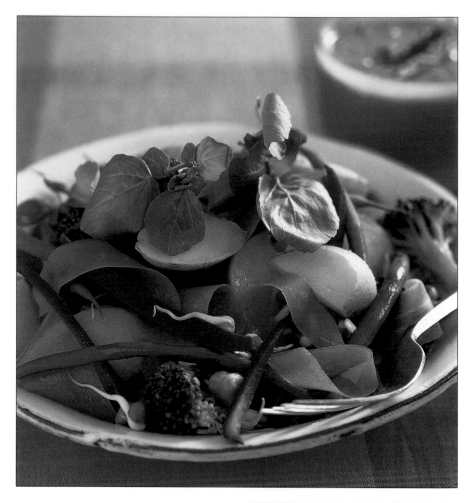

1 First make the peanut sauce. Heat the oil in a saucepan, add the chilli and garlic, and cook for 1 minute or until softened. Add the spices and cook for 1 minute. Stir in the peanut butter and water, then cook for 2 minutes until combined, stirring constantly.

2 Add the soy sauce, ginger, sugar, lime juice and coconut milk, then cook over a low heat until smooth and heated through, stirring frequently. Transfer to a bowl.

3 Bring a saucepan of lightly salted water to the boil, add the potatoes and cook for 10–15 minutes, until tender. Drain, then halve or thickly slice the potatoes, depending on their size.

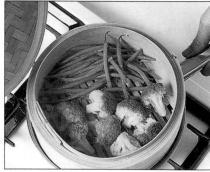

4 Meanwhile, steam the broccoli and green beans for 4–5 minutes until tender but still crisp. Add the carrots 2 minutes before the end of the cooking time.

5 Arrange the cooked vegetables on a serving platter with the red pepper and sprouted beans. Garnish with watercress and serve with the peanut sauce.

Avocado, Red Onion and Spinach Salad with Polenta Croûtons

THE SIMPLE LEMON DRESSING gives a boost of vitamin C and a sharp tang to the creamy avocado, sweet red onions and crisp spinach. Golden polenta croûtons add a delicious and healthy contrast.

INGREDIENTS

1 large red onion, cut into wedges
300g/11oz ready-made polenta, cut into
  1cm/½in cubes
olive oil, for brushing
225g/8oz baby spinach leaves
1 avocado, peeled, stoned and sliced
5ml/1 tsp lemon juice

For the dressing
60ml/4 tbsp extra virgin olive oil
juice of ½ lemon
salt and freshly ground black pepper
Serves 4

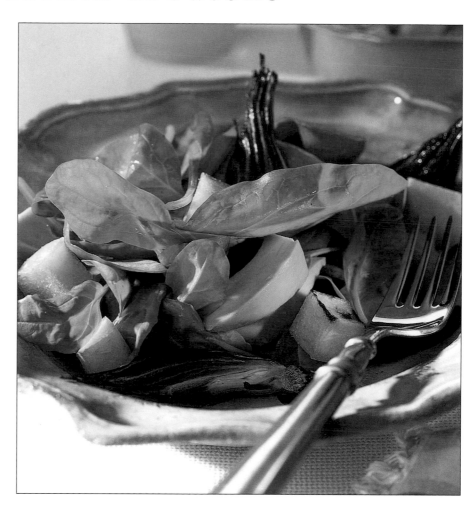

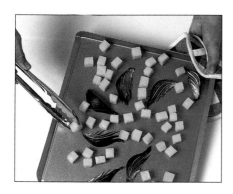

1 Preheat the oven to 200°C/400°F/ Gas 6. Place the onion wedges and polenta cubes on a lightly oiled baking sheet and bake for 25 minutes or until the onion is tender and the polenta is crisp and golden, turning them regularly to prevent them sticking. Leave to cool slightly.

2 Meanwhile, make the dressing. Place the olive oil, lemon juice and seasoning to taste in a bowl or screw-top jar. Stir or shake thoroughly to combine.

3 Place the baby spinach leaves in a serving bowl. Toss the avocado slices in the lemon juice to prevent them browning, then add to the spinach with the roasted onions.

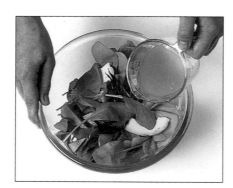

4 Pour the dressing over the salad and toss gently to combine. Sprinkle the polenta croûtons on top or hand them round separately and serve immediately.

HEALTH BENEFITS

Avocados have been traditionally regarded as a high fat food that should be avoided. However, although they do contain high amounts of fat, it is beneficial monounsaturated fat, and new research has revealed that regularly eating avocados can actually decrease the level of cholesterol in the body. Avocados also have a valuable mineral content and eating them can improve the condition of your skin and hair.

COOK'S TIP

If you can't find ready-made polenta, you can make your own using instant polenta grains. Simply cook according to the packet instructions, then pour into a tray and leave to cool and set.

White Bean Salad with Roasted Red Pepper Dressing

THE SPECKLED HERB AND RED pepper dressing adds a wonderful colour contrast to this wholesome and nutritious salad. This dish offers a good supply of low-fat protein and is rich in vitamins and minerals.

INGREDIENTS

1 large red pepper
60ml/4 tbsp olive oil
1 large garlic clove, crushed
25g/1oz/1 cup fresh oregano leaves or
*   flat leaf parsley*
15ml/1 tbsp balsamic vinegar
400g/14oz/3 cups canned flageolet beans,
*   drained and rinsed*
200g/7oz/1 ½ cups canned cannellini
*   beans, drained and rinsed*
salt and freshly ground black pepper
Serves 4

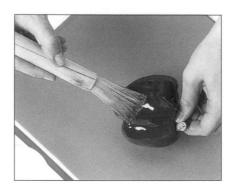

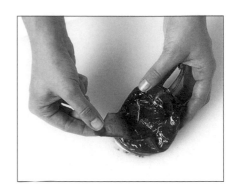

1 Preheat the oven to 200°C/400°F/ Gas 6. Place the red pepper on a baking sheet, brush with oil and roast for 30 minutes or until the skin wrinkles and the flesh is soft.

2 Remove the pepper from the oven and place in a plastic bag. Seal and leave to cool. (This makes the skin easier to remove.)

3 When the pepper is cool enough to handle, remove it from the bag and peel off the skin. Rinse under cold running water. Slice the pepper in half, remove the seeds and dice. Set aside.

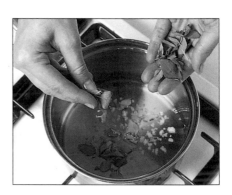

4 Heat the remaining oil in a saucepan and cook the garlic for 1 minute until softened. Remove from the heat, then add the oregano or parsley, the red pepper and any juices, and the balsamic vinegar.

5 Put the beans in a large bowl and pour over the dressing. Season to taste, then stir gently until combined. Serve warm.

HEALTH BENEFITS

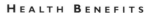

Low in fat and high in fibre and protein, pulses such as cannellini beans should be a regular part of a healthy balanced diet. They are also a good source of many minerals, including iron, potassium phosphorus and magnesium, as well as B complex vitamins.

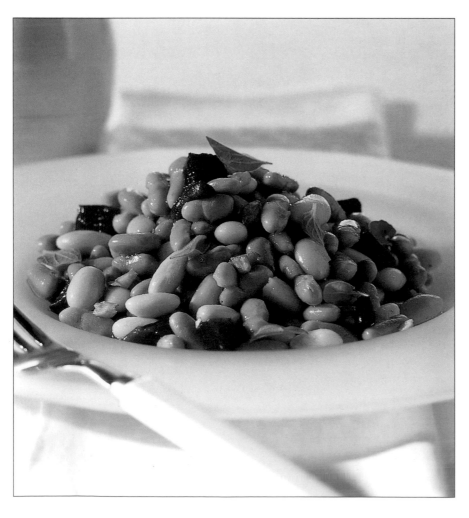

Roasted Beetroot with Horseradish Dressing

ROASTING THIS powerful cancer-fighting vegetable, gives it a delicious sweet flavour, which contrasts wonderfully with the sharp and tangy dressing.

INGREDIENTS

450g/1lb baby beetroot, preferably
   with leaves
15ml/1 tbsp olive oil

For the dressing
30ml/2 tbsp lemon juice
30ml/2 tbsp mirin
120ml/8 tbsp olive oil
30ml/2 tbsp creamed horseradish
salt and freshly ground black pepper
Serves 4

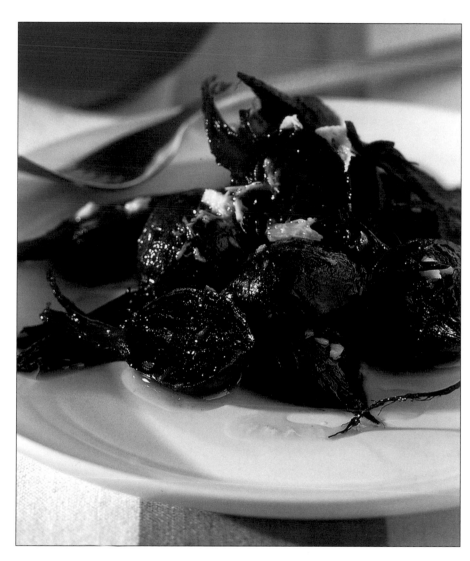

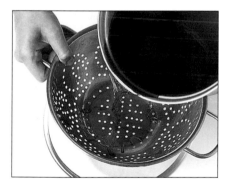

1 Cook the beetroot in boiling salted water for 30 minutes. Drain, add the olive oil and toss gently. Preheat the oven to 200°C/400°F/Gas 6.

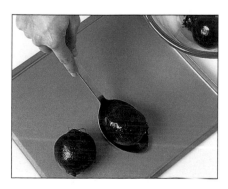

2 Place the beetroot on a baking sheet and roast for 40 minutes or until tender when pierced with a knife.

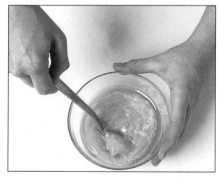

3 Meanwhile, make the dressing. Whisk together the lemon juice, mirin, olive oil and horseradish until smooth and creamy. Season.

4 Cut the beetroot in half, place in a bowl and add the dressing. Toss gently and serve immediately.

HEALTH BENEFITS

Beetroot has a reputation for containing cancer-fighting compounds and is thought to enhance the immune system. It is a powerful blood-purifier and is rich in iron, vitamins C and A, and folates, which are essential for healthy cells.

COOK'S TIP

This salad is probably at its best served warm, but you can make it in advance, if you wish, and serve it at room temperature. Add the dressing to the beetroot just before serving.

Watercress, Pear, Walnut and Roquefort Salad

PEPPERY WATERCRESS LEAVES combine wonderfully with sweet pears and crunchy walnuts to pack a powerful healing punch.

INGREDIENTS

75g/3oz/1/2 cup shelled walnuts, halved
2 red Williams pears, cored and sliced
15ml/1 tbsp lemon juice
150g/5oz/1 large bunch watercress, tough
  stalks removed
200g/7oz/scant 2 cups Roquefort cheese,
  cut into chunks

For the dressing
45ml/3 tbsp extra virgin olive oil
30ml/2 tbsp lemon juice
2.5ml/1/2 tsp clear honey
5ml/1 tsp Dijon mustard
salt and freshly ground black pepper
Serves 4

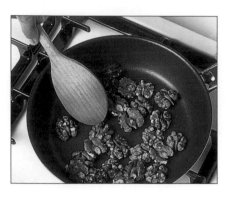

1 Toast the walnuts in a dry frying pan for 2 minutes until golden, tossing frequently to prevent them burning.

HEALTH BENEFITS

Watercress is reputed to energize the liver, kidney and bladder. It provides vitamins A and C, thought to play a role in combating cancer. It also contains natural antibiotic compounds.

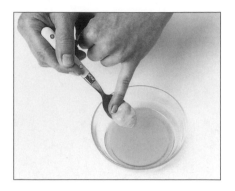

2 Meanwhile, make the dressing. Place the olive oil, lemon juice, honey, mustard and seasoning in a bowl or screw-top jar. Stir or shake thoroughly to combine.

3 Toss the pear slices in the lemon juice, then place them in a bowl and add the watercress, walnuts and Roquefort. Pour the dressing over the salad, toss well and serve immediately.

Panzanella

OPEN-TEXTURED, ITALIAN-STYLE bread and fresh vegetables combine to produce a healthful and invigorating light lunch.

INGREDIENTS

275g/10oz/10 slices day-old Italian-style
  bread, thickly sliced
1 cucumber, peeled and cut into chunks
5 tomatoes, seeded and diced
1 large red onion, chopped
200g/7oz/1 1/3 cups good quality olives
20 basil leaves, torn

For the dressing
60ml/4 tbsp extra virgin olive oil
15ml/1 tbsp red or white wine vinegar
salt and freshly ground black pepper
Serves 6

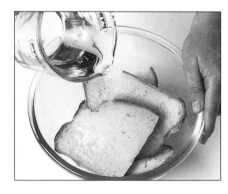

1 Soak the bread in water for about 2 minutes, then lift out and squeeze gently, first with your hands and then in a dish towel to remove any excess water. Chill for 1 hour.

HEALTH BENEFITS

Rich in healthy monounsaturated fat, olives act as a gentle laxative and have a soothing effect on the digestive system.

2 Meanwhile, to make the dressing, place the oil, vinegar and seasoning in a bowl or screw-top jar. Shake or mix thoroughly to combine. Place the cucumber, tomatoes, onion and olives in a bowl.

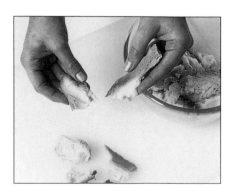

3 Break the bread into chunks and add to the bowl with the basil. Pour the dressing over the salad, and toss before serving.

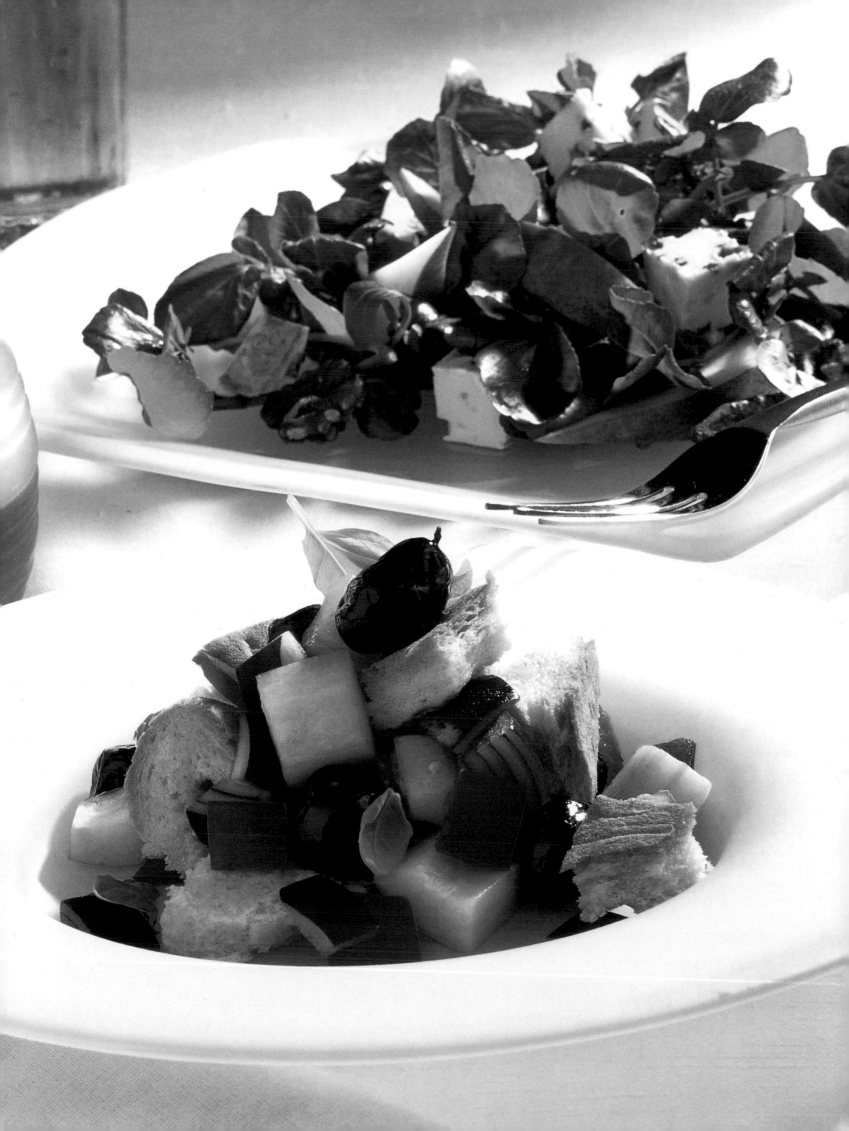

Fresh Tuna Salad Niçoise

NUTRIENT-RICH OILY FISH and fresh salad vegetables make the perfect combination for a summer lunch.

INGREDIENTS

4 tuna steaks, about 150g/5oz each
30ml/2 tbsp olive oil
225g/8oz fine French beans, trimmed
1 small cos lettuce or 2 Little Gem lettuces
4 new potatoes, boiled
4 ripe tomatoes, or 12 cherry tomatoes
2 red peppers, seeded and cut into
    thin strips
4 hard-boiled eggs, sliced
8 drained anchovy fillets in oil,
    halved lengthways
16 large black olives
salt and ground black pepper
12 fresh basil leaves, to garnish

For the dressing

15ml/1 tbsp red wine vinegar
90ml/6 tbsp olive oil
1 fat garlic clove, crushed
Serves 4

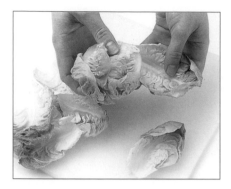

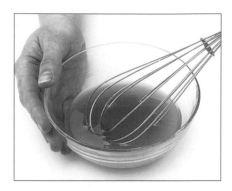

3 Separate the lettuce leaves and wash and dry them. Arrange them on four individual serving plates. Slice the potatoes and tomatoes, if large, (leave cherry tomatoes whole) and divide them among the plates. Arrange the French beans and strips of red pepper over them.

4 Shell the hard-boiled eggs and cut them into thick slices. Place two half eggs on each plate with an anchovy fillet draped over. Scatter four olives on to each plate.

5 To make the dressing, whisk together the vinegar, olive oil and garlic and season to taste. Drizzle over the salads, arrange the tuna steaks on top, scatter over the basil and serve.

HEALTH BENEFITS

Tuna is an oily fish, which makes it a good source of omega-3 fatty acids. These have been found to play a crucial role in reducing the risk of heart disease. Just one serving of oily fish a week is said to reduce the risk of heart attack.

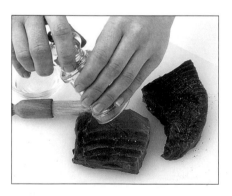

1 Brush the tuna on both sides with a little olive oil and season with salt and pepper. Heat a ridged griddle or the grill until very hot, then grill the tuna steaks for 1–2 minutes on each side; the flesh should still be pink and juicy in the middle. Set aside.

2 Cook the beans in a saucepan of lightly salted boiling water for 4–5 minutes or until crisp-tender. Drain, refresh under cold water and drain well again.

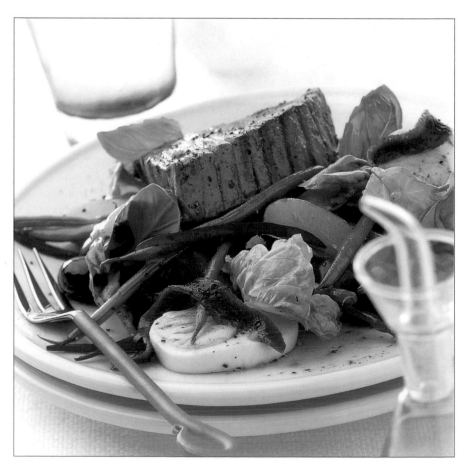

Piquant Prawn Salad

INGREDIENTS

200g/7oz rice vermicelli or stir-fry
   rice noodles

8 baby corn cobs, halved

150g/5oz mangetouts

15ml/1 tbsp stir-fry oil

2 garlic cloves, finely chopped

2.5cm/1in piece fresh root ginger, peeled
   and finely chopped

1 fresh red or green chilli, seeded and
   finely chopped

450g/1lb raw peeled tiger prawns

4 spring onions, very thinly sliced

15ml/1 tbsp sesame seeds, toasted

1 lemon grass stalk, thinly shredded,
   to garnish

For the dressing

15ml/1 tbsp snipped chives

15ml/1 tbsp nam pla (Thai fish sauce)

5ml/1 tsp soy sauce

45ml/3 tbsp groundnut oil

5ml/1 tsp sesame oil

30ml/2 tbsp rice vinegar

Serves 4

1 Put the rice vermicelli or noodles in a wide heatproof bowl, pour over boiling water and leave for 5 minutes. Drain, refresh under cold water and drain again. Tip back into the bowl and set aside until required.

2 Boil or steam the corn cobs and mangetouts for about 3 minutes; they should still be crunchy. Refresh under cold water and drain. Make the dressing. Put the chives, nam pla, soy sauce, groundnut oil, sesame oil and rice vinegar in a screw-top jar, close tightly and shake well to combine.

HEALTH BENEFITS

Prawns provide an excellent supply of B vitamins, which promote a healthy glowing complexion and combat dry skin. These vitamins also play a crucial role in how the body copes with stressful situations, and are said to help in fighting insomnia.

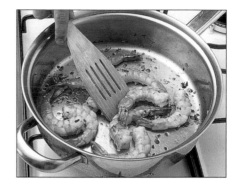

3 Heat the oil in a large frying pan or wok. Add the garlic, ginger and chilli and cook for 1 minute. Add the tiger prawns and stir-fry for about 3 minutes, until they have just turned pink. Stir in the spring onions, corn cobs, mangetouts and sesame seeds, and toss lightly to mix.

4 Tip the contents of the pan or wok over the rice vermicelli or noodles. Pour the dressing on top and toss well. Serve immediately, garnished with lemon grass. Alternatively, chill for an hour before serving.

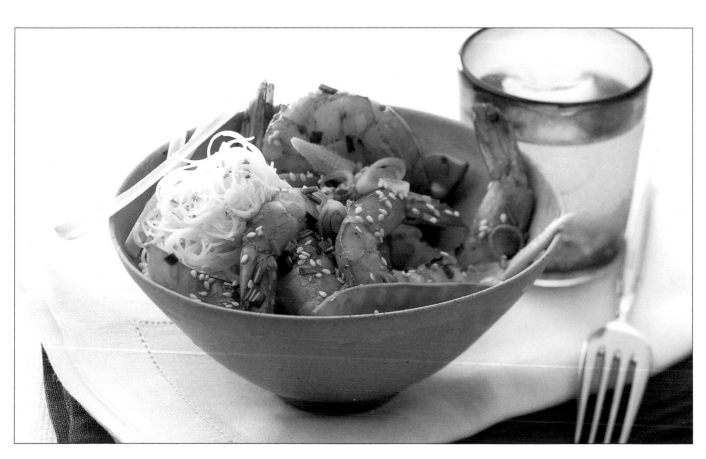

Rosemary and Garlic Roasted New Potatoes

FRESH ROSEMARY and lots of garlic give these delicious little potatoes an extra healing boost.

INGREDIENTS

800g/1³/4lb small new potatoes
5 garlic cloves, peeled and bruised
3 sprigs of rosemary
30ml/2 tbsp olive oil
sea salt and freshly ground black pepper
Serves 4

HEALTH BENEFITS

So much can be said about the healing power of garlic. It is particularly valued for its ability to boost the immune system. As a result, it has been found to be helpful in treating AIDS patients.

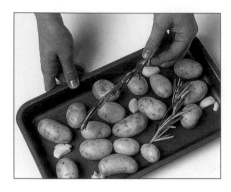

I Preheat the oven to 200°C/400°F/ Gas 6. Put the potatoes, garlic and rosemary in a roasting tin. Add the oil and toss to coat. Season well.

VARIATION

Shallots can be roasted in the same way. Cook for 35 minutes or until tender.

2 Bake for 40–45 minutes until the potatoes are crisp on the outside and soft in the centre.

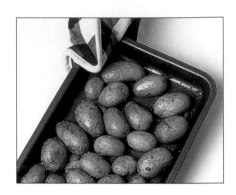

3 Remove the tin from the oven halfway through cooking and shake the tin to turn the potatoes and coat them in oil. Discard the rosemary and garlic, if you wish, and serve hot.

Honey-glazed Carrots

NATURALLY SWEET CARROTS, sautéed in a glossy honey and mustard glaze, are rich in antioxidants and make the perfect addition to any meal.

INGREDIENTS

450g/1lb/2¹/2 cups carrots, cut into
    thick matchsticks
25g/1oz/2 tbsp butter
15ml/1 tbsp olive oil
1 garlic clove, crushed
15ml/1 tbsp chopped fresh rosemary leaves
5ml/1 tsp Dijon mustard
10ml/2 tsp clear honey
Serves 4

COOK'S TIP

Other root vegetables, such as parsnips, celeriac, baby turnips and swede can be cooked in this honey glaze. Buy organic vegetables whenever possible and simply scrub, or peel very thinly.

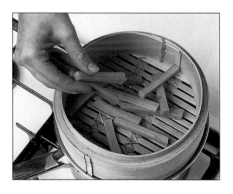

I Steam the carrots over a saucepan of boiling water for 2–4 minutes until just tender.

HEALTH BENEFITS

Carrots are a good source of beta-carotene, the plant form of vitamin A (just one carrot supplies enough of this vitamin for an entire day). A deficiency of vitamin A leads to night blindness, so the old saying that carrots help you see in the dark may be based on fact.

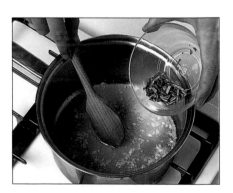

2 Heat the butter and oil in a heavy-based saucepan, add the garlic and rosemary and cook, stirring, for 1 minute or until the garlic is golden brown.

3 Add the carrots, mustard and honey to the pan, and cook, stirring constantly, for 2 minutes or until the carrots are only just tender. Serve immediately.

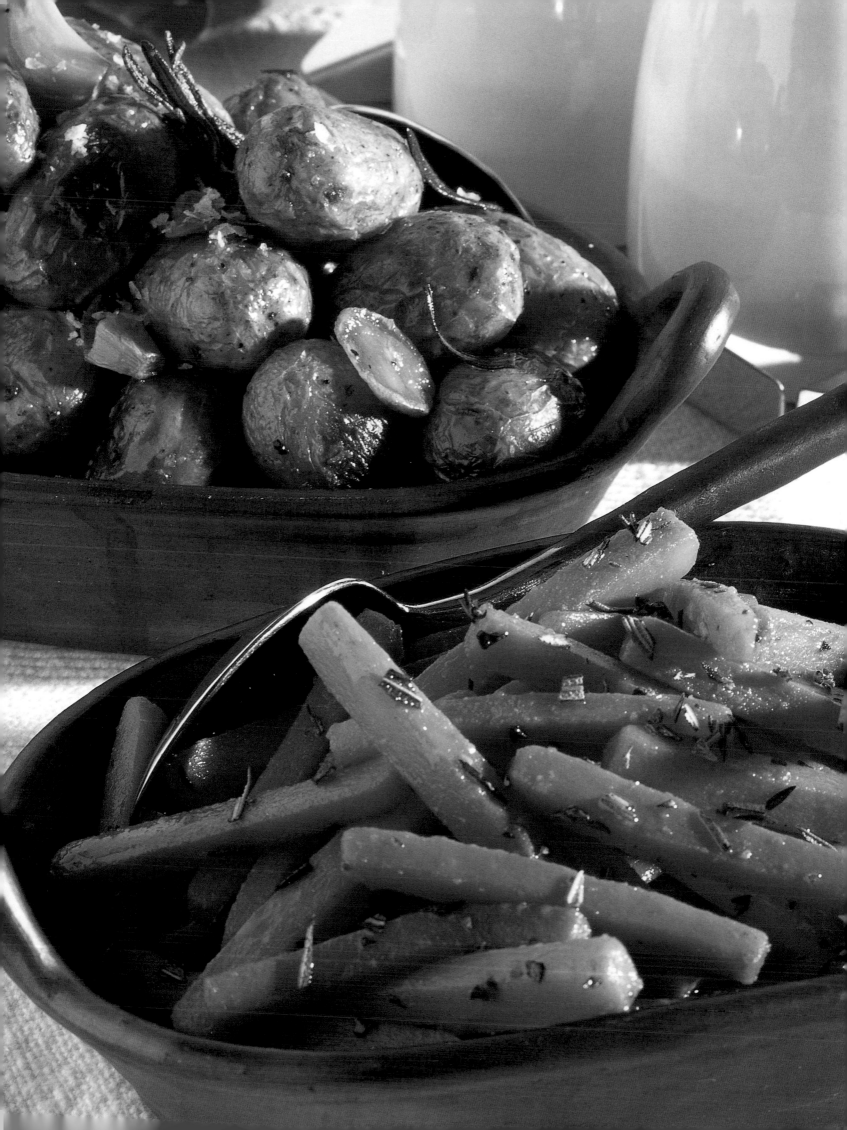

Courgettes in Rich Tomato Sauce

IN MEDITERRANEAN countries, where the ingredients used in this richly-flavoured dish are eaten as part of the staple diet, there is a much lower incidence of heart disease and cancer.

INGREDIENTS

15ml/1 tbsp olive oil
1 onion, chopped
1 garlic clove, chopped
4 courgettes, thickly sliced
400g/14oz/3 cups canned tomatoes, strained
2 tomatoes, peeled, seeded and chopped
5ml/1 tsp vegetable bouillon powder
15ml/1 tbsp tomato purée
salt and freshly ground black pepper
Serves 4

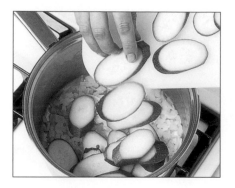

1 Heat the oil in a heavy-based saucepan, add the onion and garlic and sauté for 5 minutes or until the onion is softened, stirring occasionally. Add the courgettes and cook for a further 5 minutes.

VARIATION

Add 1 or 2 sliced and seeded red peppers with the courgettes in step 1.

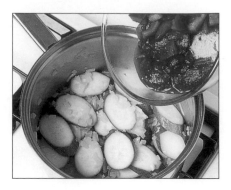

2 Add the canned and fresh tomatoes, bouillon powder and tomato purée. Stir well, then simmer for 10–15 minutes until the sauce is thickened and the courgettes are just tender. Season to taste and serve.

HEALTH BENEFITS

Like carrots, courgettes are a good source of both betacarotene and vitamin C.

Baked Fennel with a Crumb Crust

FENNEL, with its hint of aniseed, makes a delicious partner to all sorts of pasta dishes, and is said to have natural healing qualities.

INGREDIENTS

3 fennel bulbs, cut lengthways into quarters
30ml/2 tbsp olive oil
1 garlic clove, chopped
50g/2oz/1 cup day-old wholemeal breadcrumbs
30ml/2 tbsp chopped fresh flat leaf parsley
salt and freshly ground black pepper
fennel leaves, to garnish (optional)
Serves 4

VARIATION

To make a cheese-topped version of this dish, add 60ml/4 tbsp finely grated strong-flavoured cheese, such as mature Cheddar, Red Leicester or Parmesan, to the breadcrumb mixture in step 3.

1 Cook the fennel in a saucepan of boiling salted water for 10 minutes or until just tender.

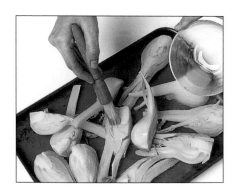

2 Drain the fennel and place in a baking dish or roasting tin, then brush with half of the olive oil. Preheat the oven to 190°C/375°F/Gas 5.

HEALTH BENEFITS

A natural diuretic, fennel is also known for its ability to relieve wind and flatulence.

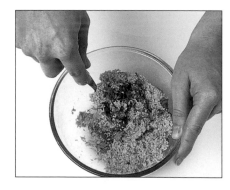

3 In a small bowl, mix together the garlic, breadcrumbs and parsley with the rest of the oil. Sprinkle the mixture evenly over the fennel, then season well.

4 Bake for 30 minutes or until the fennel is tender and the breadcrumbs are crisp and golden. Serve hot, garnished with a few fennel leaves, if you wish.

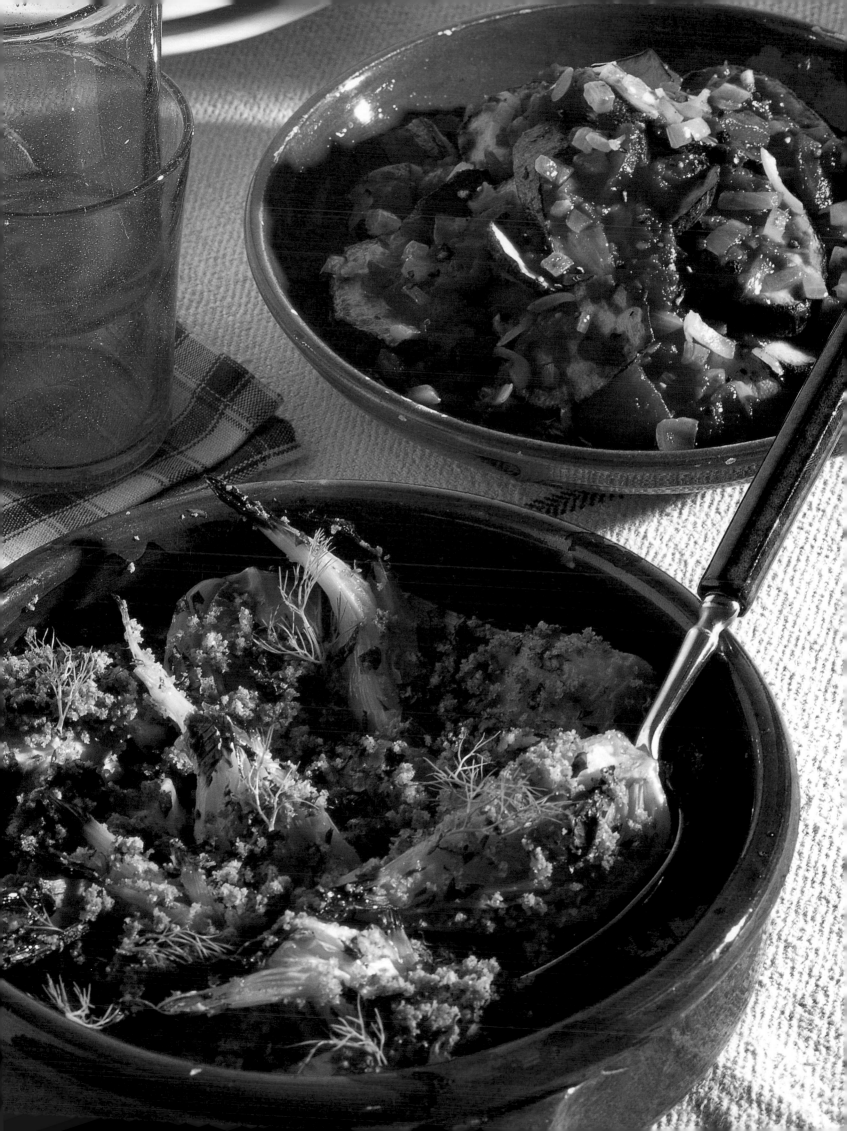

Spring Vegetable Stir-fry

FAST, FRESH AND PACKED WITH healthy vegetables, this stir-fry is delicious served with marinated tofu and rice or noodles.

INGREDIENTS

15ml/1 tbsp groundnut or vegetable oil
5ml/1 tsp toasted sesame oil
1 garlic clove, chopped
2.5cm/1 in piece fresh root ginger,
  finely chopped
225g/8oz baby carrots
350g/12oz/3 cups broccoli florets
175g/6oz/1/3 cup asparagus tips
2 spring onions, cut on the diagonal
175g/6oz/1 1/2 cups spring greens,
  finely shredded
30ml/2 tbsp light soy sauce
15ml/1 tbsp apple juice
15ml/1 tbsp sesame seeds, toasted
Serves 4

1 Heat a frying pan or wok over a high heat. Add the groundnut or vegetable oil and the sesame oil, and reduce the heat. Add the garlic and sauté for 2 minutes.

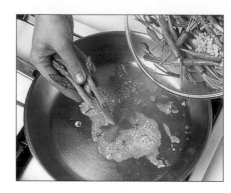

2 Add the chopped ginger, carrots, broccoli and asparagus tips to the pan and stir-fry for 4 minutes. Add the spring onions and spring greens and stir-fry for a further 2 minutes.

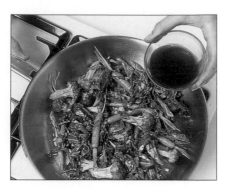

3 Add the soy sauce and apple juice and cook for 1–2 minutes until the vegetables are tender; add a little water if they appear dry. Sprinkle the sesame seeds on top and serve.

HEALTH BENEFITS

Green and orange vegetables are an excellent source of betacarotene, as well as vitamins C and E.

Oriental Green Beans

THIS IS A SIMPLE AND DELICIOUS way of enlivening green beans. The aromatic flavours of garlic and ginger add not only to its taste but also to its healing qualities.

INGREDIENTS

450g/1lb/3 cups green beans
15ml/1 tbsp olive oil
5ml/1 tsp sesame oil
2 garlic cloves, crushed
2.5cm/1 in piece fresh root ginger,
  finely chopped
30ml/2 tbsp dark soy sauce
Serves 4

VARIATION

Substitute other green beans, if you wish. Runner beans and other flat varieties should be cut diagonally into thick slices before steaming.

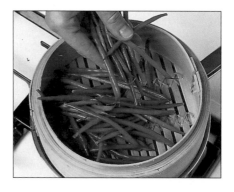

1 Steam the beans over a saucepan of boiling salted water for 4 minutes or until just tender.

HEALTH BENEFITS

• *This dish contains good amounts of garlic and fresh root ginger, both of which are said to give the immune system a significant boost.*
• *Recent studies confirm that ginger may be more effective in preventing nausea than prescribed drugs.*

2 Meanwhile, heat the olive and sesame oils in a heavy-based saucepan, add the garlic and sauté for 2 minutes.

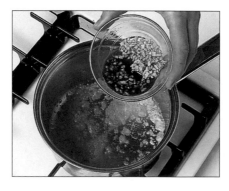

3 Stir in the ginger and soy sauce and cook, stirring constantly, for a further 2–3 minutes until the liquid has reduced, then pour this mixture over the warm beans. Leave for a few minutes to allow all the flavours to mingle before serving.

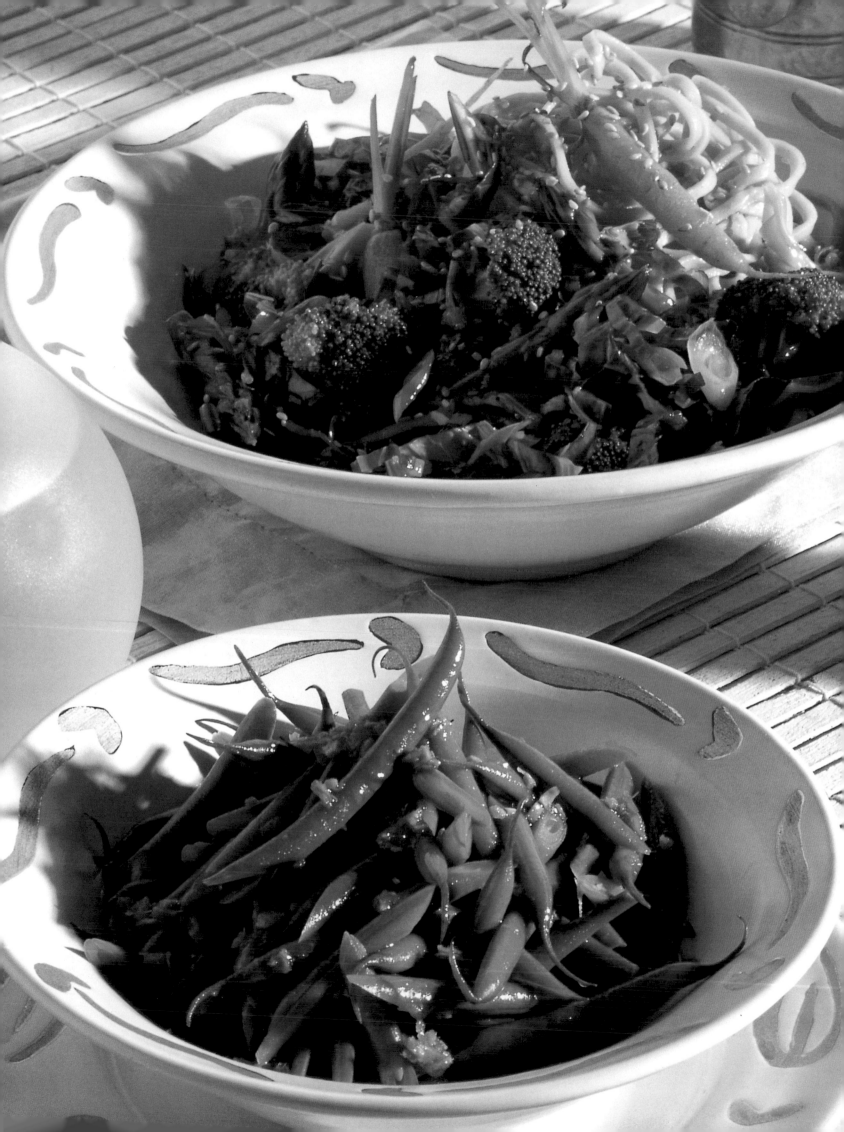

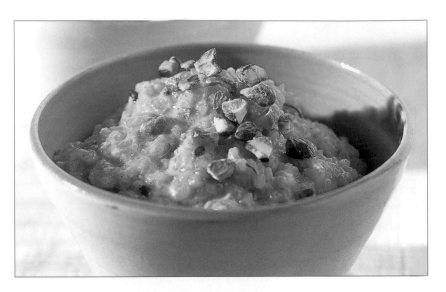

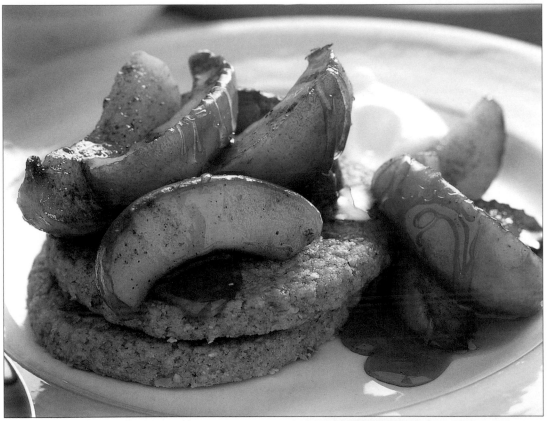

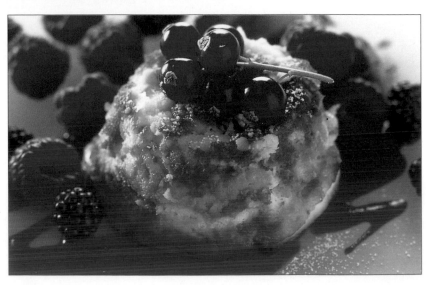

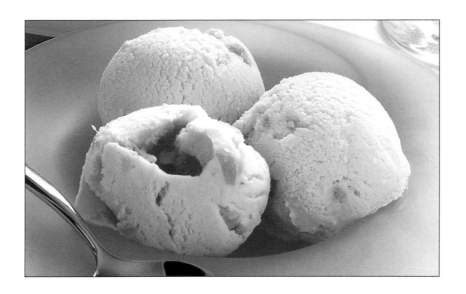

DESSERTS

Many of the delicious temptations in this chapter are as luscious as you like, but won't add to your waistline or leave you feeling unsatisfied. Delicately flavoured Mango and Orange Sorbet, and Rhubarb and Ginger Yogurt Ice are stunning examples, as are the Baked Ricotta Cakes with Red Sauce. Pan-fried Apple Slices with Walnut Shortbread taste simply wonderful, while Winter Fruit Poached in Mulled Wine makes the most of dried fruit, which contributes valuable minerals, including iron, potassium and calcium, as well as B complex vitamins and fibre.

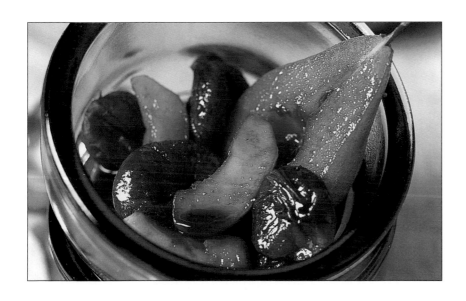

Mango and Orange Sorbet

FRESH AND TANGY, and gloriously vibrant in colour, this sorbet makes an ideal after dinner cleanser.

INGREDIENTS
115g/4oz/½ cup golden caster sugar
2 large mangoes
juice of 1 orange
1 egg white (optional)
thinly pared strips of fresh unwaxed orange
 rind, to decorate
Serves 2–4

1 Gently heat the sugar and 300ml/ ½ pint/1¼ cups water in a pan until the sugar has dissolved. Bring to the boil, then reduce the heat and simmer for 5 minutes. Leave to cool.

2 Cut away the two sides of the mangoes close to the stone. Peel, then cut the flesh from the stones. Dice the fruit and discard the stones.

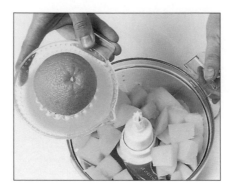

3 Process the mango flesh and orange juice in a food processor with the sugar syrup until smooth.

4 Pour the mixture into a freezer-proof container and freeze for 2 hours until semi-frozen. Whisk the egg white, if using, until it forms stiff peaks, then stir it into the sorbet. Whisk well to remove any ice crystals and freeze until solid.

5 Transfer the sorbet to the fridge 10 minutes before serving. Serve, decorated with orange rind.

HEALTH BENEFITS

Mangoes and oranges aid the digestion, boost the immune system and are said to cleanse the blood. They are also an excellent source of vitamins A and C.

Rhubarb and Ginger Yogurt Ice

YOGURT AND GINGER combine to create a soothing, digestive dessert.

INGREDIENTS
300g/11oz/scant 1½ cups set natural
 live yogurt
200g/7oz/scant 1 cup fromage frais
375g/13oz/3 cups rhubarb, trimmed
 and chopped
45ml/3 tbsp stem ginger syrup
30ml/2 tbsp clear honey
3 pieces stem ginger, finely chopped
Serves 6

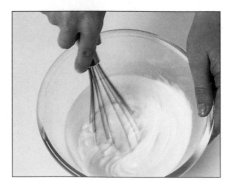

1 In a bowl, whisk together the yogurt and fromage frais.

2 Pour the yogurt mixture into a shallow freezer-proof container and freeze for 1 hour.

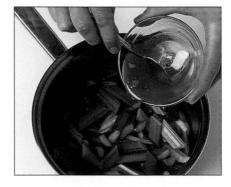

3 Meanwhile, put the rhubarb, stem ginger syrup and honey in a large saucepan and cook over a low heat for 15 minutes, or until the rhubarb is soft. Leave to cool, then purée in a food processor or blender.

4 Remove the semi-frozen yogurt mixture from the freezer and fold in the rhubarb and stem ginger purée. Beat well until smooth. Add the chopped stem ginger.

5 Return the yogurt ice to the freezer and freeze for a further 2 hours. Remove from the freezer and beat again, then freeze until solid. Serve scoops of the yogurt ice on individual plates or in bowls.

HEALTH BENEFITS

• Rhubarb is rich in potassium and is an effective laxative. However, it is also high in oxalic acid, which is reputed to inhibit the absorption of iron and calcium and can exasperate joint problems, such as arthritis. The leaves are poisonous and should never be eaten.
• Stem ginger retains many of the health-giving qualities of fresh ginger. It aids digestion and is effective in treating gastrointestinal disorders.

COOK'S TIP

Take the yogurt ice out of the freezer and transfer it to the fridge 15 minutes before serving to allow it to soften.

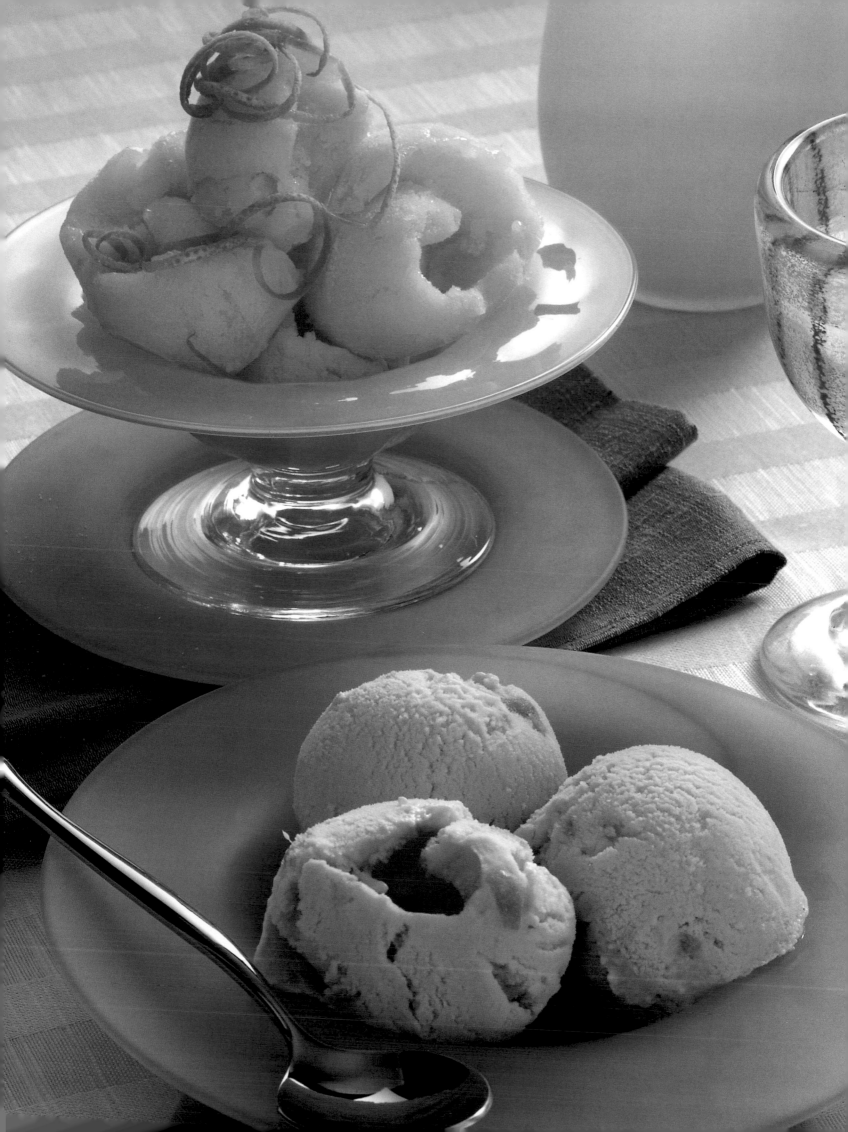

Pan-fried Apple Slices with Walnut Shortbread

SOFT, CARAMELIZED APPLES AND crisp nutty shortbread make a healthy treat with their supply of vitamins and minerals. Serve warm with a spoonful of low-fat yogurt.

INGREDIENTS

25g/1oz/2 tbsp unsalted butter
4 dessert apples, cored and thinly sliced
30ml/2 tbsp soft light brown sugar
10ml/2 tsp ground ginger
5ml/1 tsp ground cinnamon
2.5ml/1/2 tsp ground nutmeg

For the walnut shortbread

75g/3oz/2/3 cup wholemeal flour
75g/3oz/2/3 cup unbleached plain flour
25g/1oz/1/4 cup oatmeal
5ml/1 tsp baking powder
1.5ml/1/4 tsp salt
50g/2oz/1/4 cup golden caster sugar
115g/4oz/8 tbsp unsalted butter
40g/11/2oz/1/4 cup walnuts, finely chopped
15ml/1 tbsp milk, plus extra for brushing
demerara sugar, for sprinkling
Serves 4

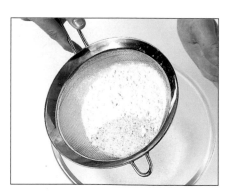

1 Preheat the oven to 180°C/350°F/ Gas 4 and grease one or two baking sheets. To make the walnut shortbread, sift together the flours, adding any bran left in the sieve, and mix with the oatmeal, baking powder, salt and sugar. Rub in the butter with your fingers until the mixture resembles fine breadcrumbs.

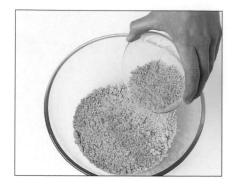

2 Add the chopped walnuts, then stir in enough of the milk to form a soft dough.

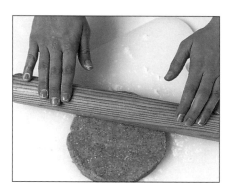

3 Gently knead the dough on a floured work surface. Form into a round, then roll out to a 5mm/1/4in thickness. Using a 7.5cm/3in fluted cutter, stamp out eight rounds – you may have some dough left over.

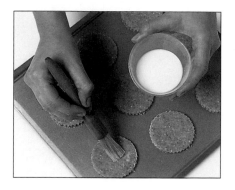

4 Place the shortbread rounds on the prepared baking sheets. Brush the tops with milk and sprinkle with sugar. Bake for 12–15 minutes until golden, then transfer to a wire rack and leave to cool.

5 To prepare the apples, melt the butter in a heavy-based frying pan. Add the apples and cook for 3–4 minutes over a gentle heat until softened. Increase the heat to medium, add the sugar and spices, and stir well. Cook for a few minutes, stirring frequently, until the sauce turns golden brown and caramelizes.

6 Place two shortbread rounds on each of four individual serving plates and spoon over the warm apples and sauce. Serve immediately.

HEALTH BENEFITS

• *Recent studies have shown that eating walnuts regularly can greatly reduce the risk of heart disease and lower the level of blood cholesterol in the body.*
• *There is much truth in the adage: "an apple a day keeps the doctor away." Apples have many health-giving properties. They help cleanse the blood, remove impurities in the liver and inhibit the growth of harmful bacteria in the digestive tract. Apples are also known to treat skin diseases and arthritis.*

COOK'S TIP

To prevent the apples browning after they are sliced, place them in a large bowl of water mixed with about 15ml/1 tbsp lemon juice.

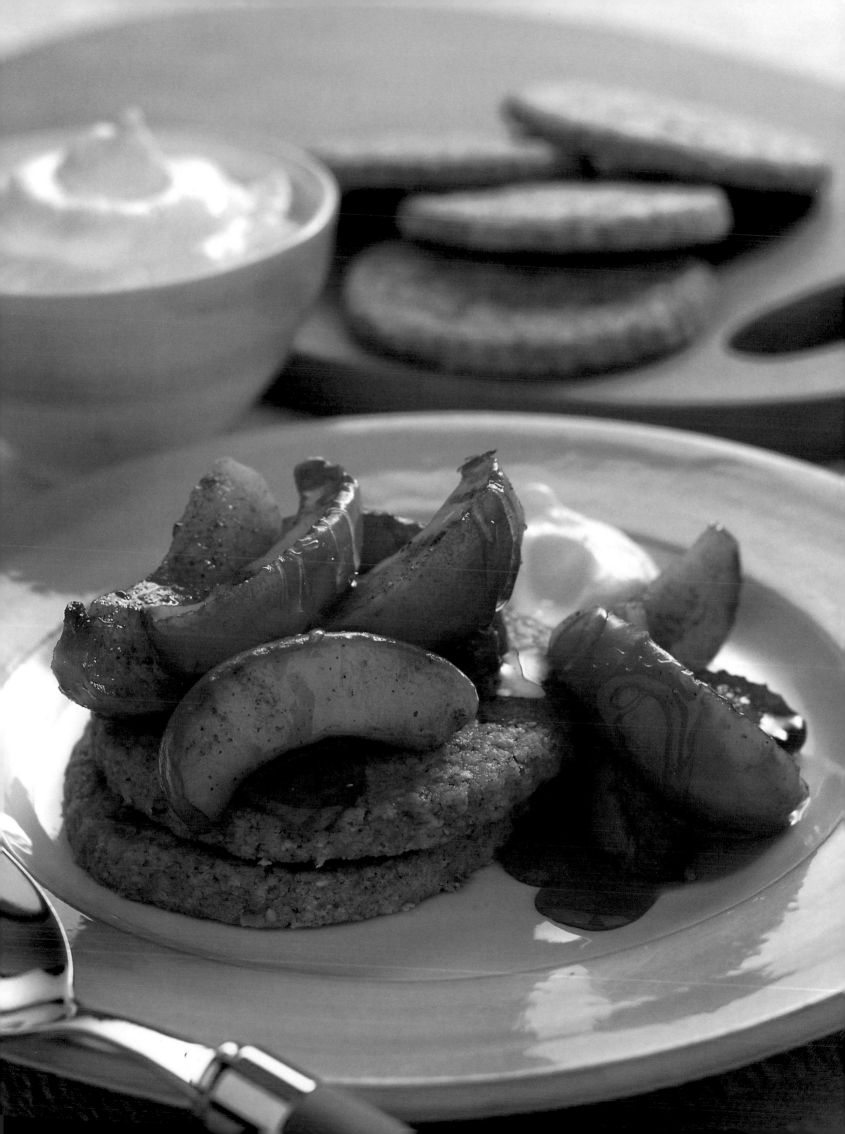

Indian Rice Pudding

THIS CREAMY PUDDING is scented with aromatic healing spices. Cardamom and nutmeg are said to aid the digestion while saffron is believed to help calm and balance the body.

INGREDIENTS

115g/4oz/³/4 cup brown short grain rice
350ml/12fl oz/1¹/2 cups boiling water
600ml/1 pint/2¹/2 cups semi-skimmed milk
6 cardamom pods, bruised
2.5ml/¹/2tsp freshly grated nutmeg
pinch of saffron strands
60ml/4 tbsp maize malt syrup
15ml/1 tbsp clear honey
50g/2oz/¹/2 cup pistachio nuts, chopped
Serves 4

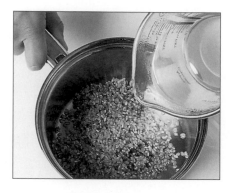

1 Wash the rice under cold running water and place in a saucepan with the boiling water. Return to the boil and boil, uncovered, for 15 minutes.

COOK'S TIP

Maize malt syrup is a natural alternative to refined sugar and can be found in health food shops.

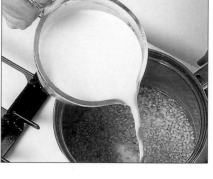

2 Pour the milk over the rice, then reduce the heat and simmer, partially covered, for 15 minutes.

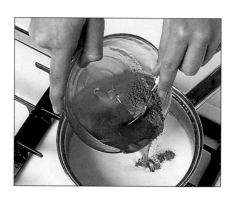

3 Add the cardamom pods, grated nutmeg, saffron, maize malt syrup and honey, and cook for a further 15 minutes, or until the rice is tender, stirring occasionally.

4 Spoon the rice into small serving bowls and sprinkle with pistachio nuts before serving hot or cold.

HEALTH BENEFITS

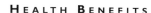

• *Brown rice is unrefined and therefore, unlike white polished rice, retains most of its fibre and nutrients. It is a source of some B complex vitamins and vitamin E.*
• *Pistachio nuts are densely packed with nourishment, being rich in protein, vitamins and minerals. However, because of their high fat content, they go rancid quickly, so buy them in a shop with a high turnover of stock and store them in a cool dry place. Due to their high fat content, pistachio nuts should be eaten in moderation.*

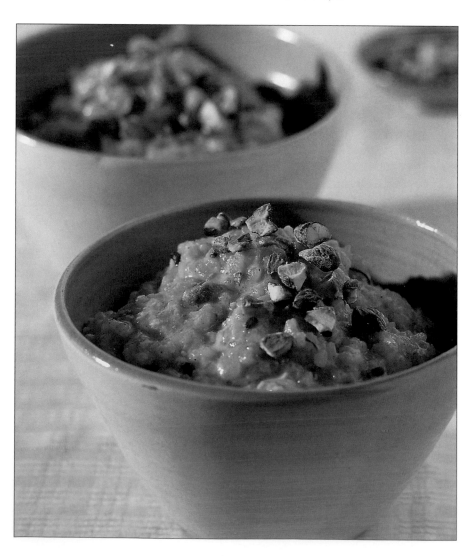

Winter Fruit Poached in Mulled Wine

FRESH APPLES AND PEARS ARE combined with dried apricots and figs to create a spicy cocktail of essential vitamins and minerals.

INGREDIENTS

300ml/½ pint/1¼ cups red wine
300ml/½ pint/1¼ cups fresh orange juice
finely grated rind and juice of 1 orange
45ml/3 tbsp clear honey or barley
    malt syrup
1 cinnamon stick, broken in half
4 cloves
4 cardamom pods, split
2 pears, such as Comice or William, peeled,
    cored and halved
8 ready-to-eat dried figs
12 ready-to-eat dried unsulphured apricots
2 eating apples, peeled, cored and
    thickly sliced

Serves 4

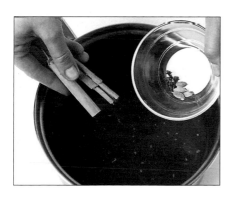

1 Put the wine, the fresh and squeezed orange juice and half the orange rind in a saucepan with the honey or syrup and spices. Bring to the boil, then reduce the heat and simmer for 2 minutes, stirring occasionally.

HEALTH BENEFITS

• *The combination of fresh and dried fruit ensures a healthy amount of vitamins and minerals, particularly of vitamin C, betacarotene, potassium and iron. The fruit is also rich in fibre.*
• *Cardamom and cinnamon soothe indigestion and, along with cloves, can offer relief from colds and coughs.*

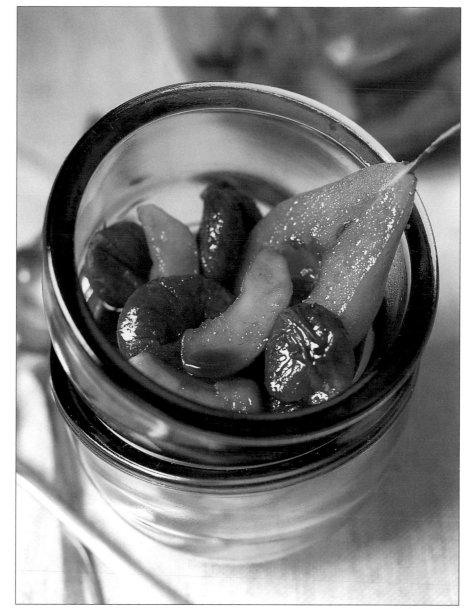

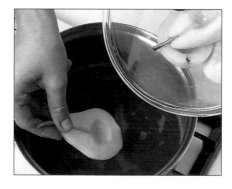

2 Add the pears, figs and apricots to the pan and cook, covered, for 25 minutes, occasionally turning the fruit in the wine mixture. Add the sliced apples and cook for a further 12–15 minutes until the fruit is tender.

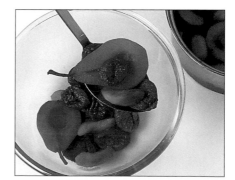

3 Remove the fruit from the pan and discard the spices. Cook the wine mixture over a high heat until reduced and syrupy, then pour it over the fruit. Serve decorated with the reserved orange rind, if wished.

Baked Ricotta Cakes with Red Sauce

THESE HONEY AND vanilla-flavoured desserts take only minutes to make and the fragrant fruity sauce adds a cancer-fighting twist.

INGREDIENTS

250g/9oz/generous 1 cup ricotta cheese
2 egg whites, beaten
60ml/4 tbsp clear honey, plus extra to taste
5ml/1 tsp vanilla essence
450g/1lb/4 cups mixed fresh or frozen
   fruit, such as strawberries, raspberries,
   blackberries and cherries
fresh mint leaves, to decorate (optional)

Serves 4

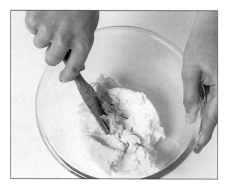

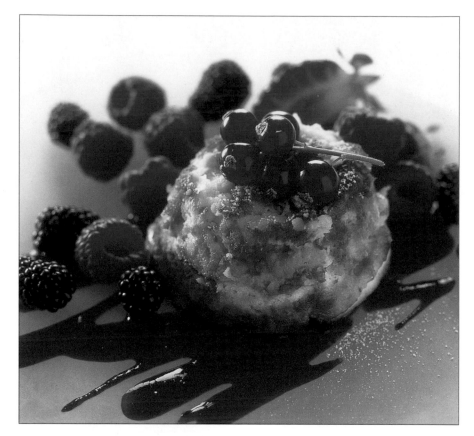

1 Preheat the oven to 180°C/350°F/ Gas 4. Place the ricotta cheese in a bowl and break it up with a wooden spoon. Add the beaten egg whites, honey and vanilla essence and mix thoroughly until the mixture is smooth and well combined.

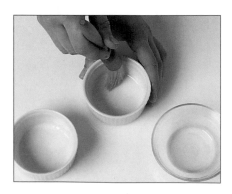

2 Lightly grease four ramekins. Spoon the ricotta mixture into the prepared ramekins and level the tops. Bake for 20 minutes or until the ricotta cakes are risen and golden.

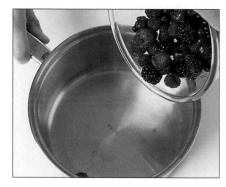

3 Meanwhile, make the fruit sauce. Reserve about a quarter of the fruit for decoration. Place the rest of the fruit in a saucepan, with a little water if the fruit is fresh, and heat gently until softened. Leave to cool slightly, remove any cherry stones, if using cherries.

COOK'S TIP

The red berry sauce can be made a day in advance. Chill until ready to use. Frozen fruit doesn't need extra water, as there are usually plenty of ice crystals clinging to the berries.

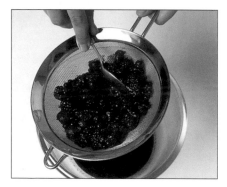

4 Press the fruit through a sieve, then taste and sweeten with honey if it is too tart. Serve the sauce, warm or cold, with the ricotta cakes. Decorate with the reserved berries and mint leaves, if using.

HEALTH BENEFITS

• Ricotta contains about 4 per cent fat, compared with 35 per cent in a hard cheese like Cheddar. It is a good source of vitamin B_{12}, calcium and protein.
• All berries are rich in the anti-cancer compound, ellagic acid, which is a powerful antioxidant.

Information File

USEFUL ADDRESSES

Australia
Australian Cancer Society
PO Box 4708
Sydney NSW 2001
Tel: (01) 2267 1944

The Biological Farmers of
  Australia Cooperative
  Ltd (BFA)
Level 1
T & G Arcade Building
477 Ruthven Street
Toowoomba QLD 4350
Tel: (07) 6393299

Diabetes Australia
National Office
5–7 Phipps Place
Deakin ACT 2615
Tel: 1 (800) 640 862

Organic Herb Growers
  of Australia (OHGA)
PO Box 6171
South Lismore NSW 2480
Tel: (02) 6622 0100

Canada
Canadian Cancer Society
10 Alcorn Avenue
Toronto
Ontario M4V 3B1
Tel: (001) 416 293 7422

Canadian Diabetic
  Association
15 Toronto Street
Suite 800
Toronto
Ontario M5C 2E3
Tel: (001) 416 363 3373

New Zealand
Cancer Society of
  New Zealand
PO Box 1724
Auckland
Tel: (09) 524 2628

South Africa
South African Diabetes
  Association
PO Box 1715
Saxonwold 21342
Tel: 011 (788) 4595

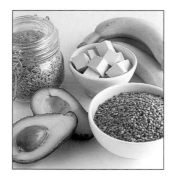

United Kingdom
Arthritis Care
18 Stephenson Way
London NW1 2HD
Tel: 020 7916 500

Arthritis Research Campaign
41 Eagle Street
London
WC1R 4AR
Tel: 01246 558033

Bacup
3 Bath Place
Rivington Street
London EC2A 3JR
Tel: 020 7613 2121

British Cancer Help Centre
Grove House
Cornwallis Grove
Clifton
Bristol BS8 4PG
Tel: 0117 980 9505

British Diabetic Association
10 Queen Anne's Street
London W1M 0BD
Tel: 020 7323 1531

British Heart Foundation
14 Fitzhardinge Street
London W1H 4DH
Tel: 020 7935 0185

British Nutrition Foundation
High Holborn House
52–54 High Holborn
London WC1V 6RQ
Tel: 020 7404 6504

Cancer Research Campaign
10 Cambridge Terrace
London NW1 4JL
Tel: 020 72241333

Gerson Therapy Information
Chapel Farm
West Humble
Dorking
Surrey RH5 6AY

Institute for Complementary
  Medicine
PO Box 194
London SE16 1QZ
Tel: 020 7237 5165

Institute for Optimum
  Nutrition
Blades Court
Deodar Road
London SW15 2NU
Tel: 020 8877 9993

Pesticides Trust
Eurolink Centre
49 Effra Road
London SW2 1BZ
Tel: 020 7274 8895

National Association
  of Health Stores
Wayside Cottage
Cuckoo Corner
Urchfont
Devizes SN10 4RA
Tel: 01380 840133

The National Osteoporosis
  Society
PO Box 10
Bath BA3 3YB
Tel: 01761 471 771

Royal Society for the
  Promotion of Health
38a St George's Drive
London SW1V 4BH
Tel: 020 7630 0121

SAFE (Sustainable Agriculture,
  Food and Environment)
  Alliance
94 White Lion Street
London N1 9PF
Tel: 020 7837 1228

The Soil Association
Bristol House
40–56 Victoria Street
Bristol BS1 6BY
Tel: 01179 290661

FURTHER READING

The Antioxidants
by Richard Passwater – Keats
Publishing Inc., Connecticut

*Fresh Vegetable and
  Fruit Juices*
by N. W. Walker – Norwalk
Press

Health Which
P.O. Box 44
Hertford SG14 1SH

Superjuice
by Michael van Straten –
Mitchell Beazley

Juicing for Health
by Caroline Wheather –
Thorsons

*The Inside Story on Food
and Health*
Subscription magazine
Berrydale Publishers
Berrydale House
5 Lawn Road
London NW3 2XS

The Optimum Nutrition Bible
by Patrick Holford – Piatkus

The Organic Directory
by Clive Lichfield – Green
Earth Books

The Sprouting Book
by Ann Wigmore – Avery
Publishing Group Inc

The Wheatgrass Book
by Ann Wigmore – Avery
Publishing Group Inc

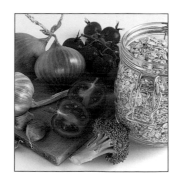

Index

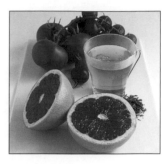
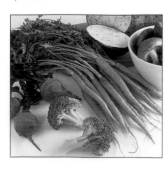

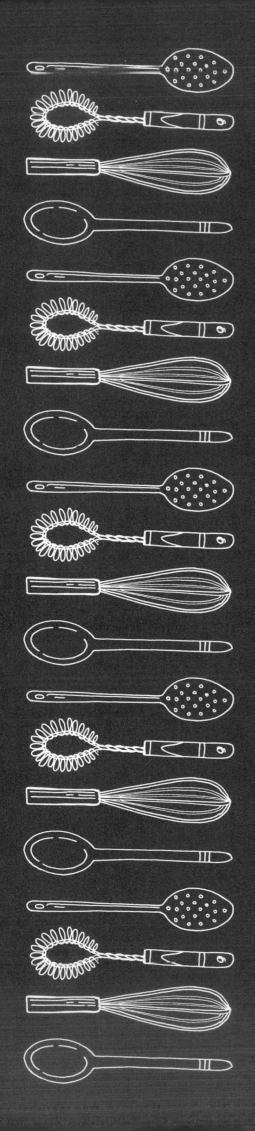